W. W. Fleischhacker and D. J. Brooks (eds.)

Stroke-Vascular Diseases

Journal of Neural Transmission
Supplement 63

SpringerWienNewYork

Prof. Dr. W. Wolfgang Fleischhacker
Department of Biological Psychiatry
Innsbruck University Clinics
Anichstrasse 35
A-6020 Innsbruck, Austria

Prof. Dr. David J. Brooks
MRC Cyclotron Unit
Hammersmith Hospital
Du Cane Road
London W12 0NN, United Kingdom

Typesetting: Best-Set Typesetter Ltd., Hong Kong

Printed on acid-free and chlorine-free bleached paper

SPIN: 10890839

CIP data applied for

With 16 Figures

ISSN 0303-6995
ISBN 3-211-83866-X (soft cover) Springer-Verlag Wien New York
ISBN 3-211-83867-8 (hard cover) Springer-Verlag Wien New York

Contents

Scott, J.: The pathogenesis of atherosclerosis and new opportunities for treatment and prevention 1
Baron, J. C.: Stroke: imaging and differential diagnosis. 19
Heiss, W.-D.: Stroke – acute interventions 37
Aichner, F., Adelwöhrer, C., Haring, H.-P.: Rehabilitation approaches to stroke 59
Kalaria, R. N., Low, W. C., Oakley, A. E., Slade, J. Y., Ince, P. G., Morris, C. M., Mizuno, T.: CADASIL and genetics of cerebral ischaemia 75
Erkinjuntti, T.: Diagnosis and management of vascular cognitive impairment and dementia 91
Ferrari, M. D., Haan, J.: The genetics of migraine: implication for treatment approaches 111
Church, S. M., Cotter, D., Bramon, E., Murray, R. M.: Does schizophrenia result from developmental or degenerative processes? 129

Listed in Current Contents/Life Sciences

J Neural Transm (2002) [Suppl] 63: 1–17

The pathogenesis of atherosclerosis and new opportunities for treatment and prevention

J. Scott

Imperial College Genetics and Genomics Research Institute, National Heart & Lung Institute, Faculty of Medicine, Imperial College of Science, Technology and Medicine, Hammersmith Campus, London, United Kingdom

Summary. Atherosclerosis is the most common disease in the industrialised world and by 2020 is predicted to be the number 1 cause of death worldwide. It is a disease of the intima and media of small to medium sized arteries that develop slowly over many years. A number of risk factors for atherosclerosis have been identified, some of these are reversible and some are not. Most prominent amongst these is an elevated level of plasma cholesterol. The lowering of cholesterol reduces the risk of heart attacks, strokes and all forms of atherosclerotic vascular disease. Nonetheless, 70% of patients go on to get symptomatic disease.

The disease process sets off an inflammatory response involving the vascular endothelium and both T and B cells of the immune system. Adhesion molecules are induced and proinflammatory cytokines and growth factors are produced by cells that orchestrate the atherosclerotic process. Narrowing the lumen of the artery leads to ischaemic symptoms. Within lesions under the influence of proteolytic enzymes released from activated macrophages (or foam cells - the hallmark of atherosclerosis) the centre of the plaque becomes liquefied to take on it's characteristic "gruel" like appearance. The shoulders of such plaque weaken and it becomes prone to rupture. Plaque rupture may lead to catastrophic thrombosis of coronary or cerebral arteries. The large amounts of tissue factor produced by macrophages make this a particularly likely event. On ulcerated plaques adherent platelets and thrombus create showers of emboli leading to ischaemic attacks.

Like the effective treatment of LDL and it's role in the prevention of ischaemic attacks there has been a move to develop new drugs that raise HDL. The discovery of the role of a new class of ABC transporter, defective in Tangiers disease, responsible for cholesterol efflux from peripheral cells including the macrophage has created great excitement around ABC1 as a drug target. New areas, new possible targets and new genetic and genomic approaches will be discussed.

Introduction

Atherosclerosis, the underlying cause of heart attacks, strokes and peripheral vascular disease, is one of the major killers in the world. By 2020 WHO statistics indicate that it will be the most common cause of morbidity and mortality in both the industrialised world and the underdeveloped world. The disease develops slowly over many years in the innermost layer of large and medium-sized arteries (Fig. 1) (Scott, 1995; Ross, 1999; Naumova and Scott, 2000; Glass and Witztum, 2001; Libby, 2001). It does not usually become manifest before the fourth of fifth decade, but then often strikes with devastating suddenness. Fifty per cent of individuals still die (25 per cent immediately) from their first heart attack; and morbidity from coronary heart disease and stroke is very significant. The disease has a profound impact on healthcare services and on industrial economies.

The lesions of atherosclerosis

Autopsy studies show that in humans atherosclerosis begins in the first and second decade of life. A similar disease can be produced in experimental animals, where diet and genetics can be manipulated to produce identical lesions. The earliest lesions are fatty streaks. These consist of an accumulation of lipid-engorged macrophages (foam cells) and T and B lymphocytes in the arterial intima. With time, the fatty streaks progress to intermediate lesions, composed of foam cells and smooth muscle cells. Advances plaques are characterised by a dense fibrous cap of connective tissues and smooth muscle cells overlying a core containing necrotic material and lipid, mainly cholesteryl esters. This material is often called gruel from the Greek athera. Cholesteryl esters may form cholesterol crystals on histological sections. Advanced plagues also contain foam cells and T and B cells, and undergo neovascularisation. This promotes plaque growth but may also provide a channel for the access of inflammatory cells and ultimately weaken the plaque.

Plaques may impede the flow of blood to an organ, giving rise to ischaemia and the symptoms of angina and intermittent claudication. Plaques that undergo denuding injury with limited thrombosis produce unstable angina or transient cerebral ischaemic attacks or deep fissuring with sudden complete occlusion of coronary artery and either stroke or myocardial infarction. The early lesions of atherosclerosis can be demonstrated by imaging modalities such as MRI, intravascular ultrasound or extra vascular B mode ultrasound, thus confirming the experience of the pathologist that lesions develop in the second decade of life.

The pathogenesis of atherosclerosis

It is now generally accepted that atherosclerosis develops as a healing response to repeated vascular–wall injury, and that risk factors (Table 1, Fig. 2)

Table 1. Risk factors for atherosclerosis

Significant genetic component	Modifiable
Elevated levels of LDL and VLDL	Yes
Low levels of HDL	Partial
Elevated lipoprotein (a)	No
Hypertension	Yes
Diabetes mellitis	Partial
Male gender	No
Elevated levels of homocysteine	Yes
Elevated levels of hemostatic factors, e.g. fibrinogen	Partial
Metabolic syndrome	Partial
Insulin resistance	Partial
Obesity	Partial
Family history	No
Environmental factors	
Smoking	Yes
Lack of exercise	Yes
High fat diet	Yes
Infectious agents	No

operate by promoting chronic cycles of damaged and repair. From the risk factors identified, the most prominent are elevated levels of LDL and VLDL. These and other risk factors shown in the table have a significant genetic component. Others are purely environmental. Many of these risk factors can be modified so that early intervention of those at risk is par-excellence the best mode of preventing atherosclerosis.

The role of cholesterol in the pathogenesis of atherosclerosis has been demonstrated by huge epidemiological studies such as the Mr Fit study in which one third of a million Americans were examined for total mortality and mortality due to cholesterol level or blood pressure (Stamler et al., 1986). There was a linear relationship between mortality and death at all levels of cholesterol. Studies on Mendelian disorders leading to very high levels of cholesterol such as familial hypercholesterolaemia tell a similar story. Comparative epidemiology and migration studies between underdeveloped countries such as China or countries like Japan where the intake of dietary cholesterol and saturated fat is low show a very low prevalence of atherosclerotic disease. Migration to the industrialised West and the adoption of the dietary habits of the West lead to an atherosclerosis risk, comparable to that in the new home countries such as the United States and the United Kingdom and Europe.

Transport and metabolism of cholesterol and triglyceride

Both cholesterol and triglyceride are absorbed from the diet and the chylomicron particle with apolipoprotein (apo)B48 as its core protein component (Fig. 3). In the circulation, this particle delivers fatty acids to peripheral fat

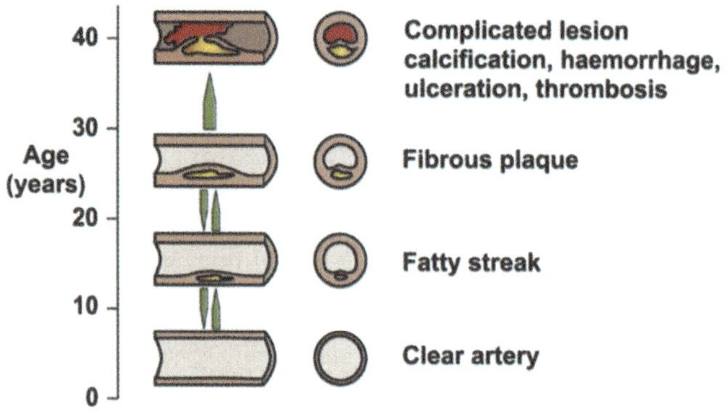

Fig. 1. Atherogenesis. Figure is a cartoon of the progression of atherosclerosis the many years until it's first catastrophic clinical manifestation

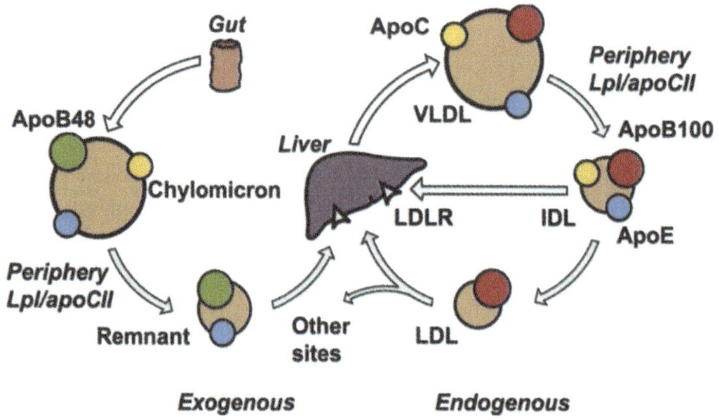

Fig. 3. Apolipoprotein B-metabolism. The figure denotes the endogenous cycle of lipoprotein metabolism with the absorption of lipids and cholesterol from the gut and the endogenous cycle of liver derived lipoproteins and LDL

Fig. 2. Atherogenesis. **a** Fatty Streak Lesion. LDL is oxidatively motivated in the intima, from minimally modified LDL (mmLDL), to extensively oxidized LDL (oxLDL). Monocytes adhere to endothelial cells. Adhesion molecules and proinflammatory cytokines are induced. Adherent monocytes migrate into the intima and differentiate into macrophages. The uptake of oxLDL by scavenger receptors produces foam cells. OxLDL cholesterol is esterified for storage or exported to extracellular HDL acceptors by cholesterol transporters, such as ABC-A1. **b** Lesion Progression. The interactions between foam cells, Th1 and Th2 cells establish a chronic inflammatory response. Lymphocytes and macrophages cytokines exert both pro- and antiatherogenic effects on the cells of the vessel wall (Fig. 4). Smooth muscle cells migrate from the medial portion of the arterial wall, proliferate and secrete extracellular matrix proteins that form a fibrous plaque. **c** Plaque Rupture and Thrombosis. Necrosis of foam cells leads to the formation of a necrotic core of extracellular cholesterol. Macrophage secretion of matrix metalloproteinases and neovascularization weaken the fibrous plaque. Plaque rupture exposes tissue factor, initiating coagulation and the formation of a thrombus (after Glass and Witzum, 2001)

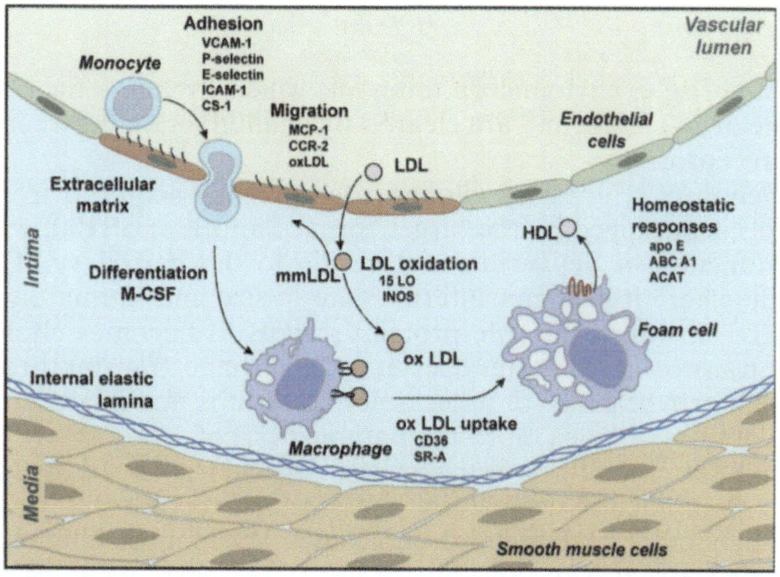
Adhesion
VCAM-1
P-selectin
E-selectin
ICAM-1
CS-1
Vascular lumen
Monocyte
Migration
MCP-1
CCR-2
oxLDL
Endothelial cells
LDL
Extracellular matrix
Homeostatic responses
apo E
ABC A1
ACAT
HDL
Intima
LDL oxidation
15 LO
iNOS
mmLDL
Differentiation
M-CSF
Foam cell
ox LDL
Internal elastic lamina
ox LDL uptake
CD36
SR-A
Macrophage
Media
Smooth muscle cells

a

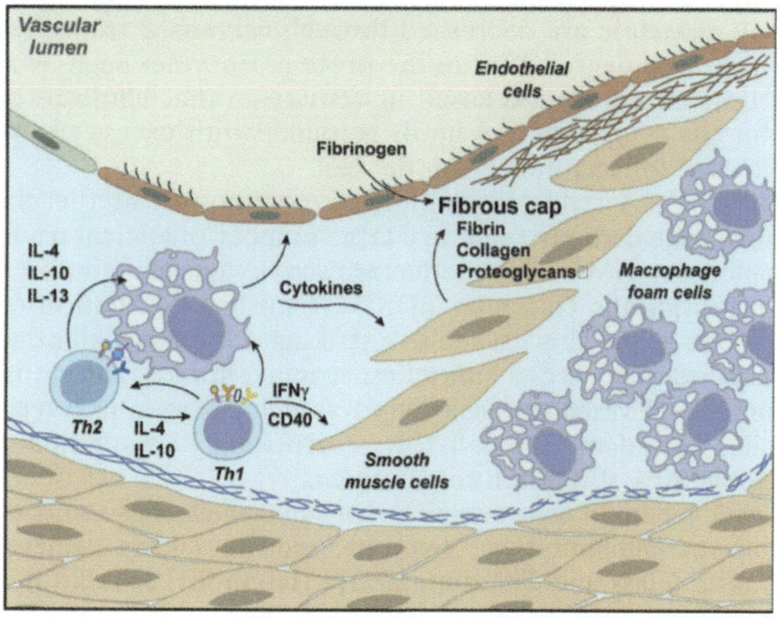
Vascular lumen
Endothelial cells
Fibrinogen
Fibrous cap
Fibrin
Collagen
Proteoglycans
IL-4
IL-10
IL-13
Macrophage foam cells
Cytokines
IFNγ
CD40
Th2
IL-4
IL-10
Th1
Smooth muscle cells

b

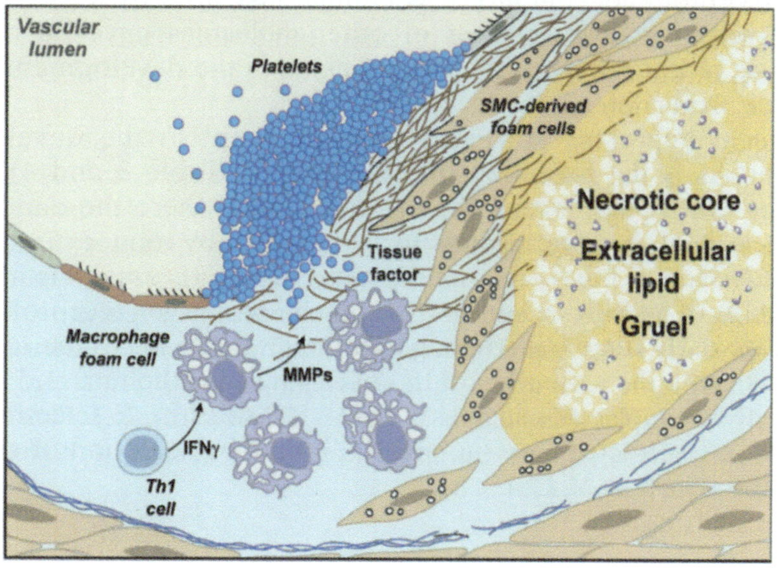
Vascular lumen
Platelets
SMC-derived foam cells
Necrotic core
Extracellular lipid
'Gruel'
Tissue factor
Macrophage foam cell
MMPs
IFNγ
Th1 cell

c

depots giving rise to chylomicron remnants which circlulate back to the liver over a time of 2–3 hours and are cleared by an interaction between apoE and the LDL receptor.

Endogenously synthesised cholesterol and some acquired from remnant lipoproteins is packaged by the larger form of apoB, apoB100, which serves a similar function of delivering triglyceride to the periphery. This shrinks the particle where it becomes intermediate in size and ultimately shrinks to become LDL in which the sole protein is apoB. It becomes cholesterol enriches by transfer of cholesteryl ester by a specific transfer protein. LDL is the "agent provocateur" of atherosclerosis. If it is not cleared by the LDL receptor pathway, it leads on to the pathogenesis of atherosclerosis.

Intracellular cholesterol homeostasis, particularly in the liver, is tightly regulated. An uptake of cholesterol by the LDL receptor pathway is limited by the availability of LDL receptor molecules. When intracellular cholesterol levels are high, enzymes responsible for the biosynthesis of cholesterol such as HMG Co A reductase are decreased through decreased transcription of the gene and increased degradation of the protein. Enzymes such as acyl cholesterol acyl transferase are increased in activity so that cholesterol ester can be stored in the cytoplasm and apoB is loaded with excess triglyceride and cholesteryl ester for secretion from the cell.

The HMG Co-A reductase inhibitors, now known as the class of drug called statins, have demonstrated in a large number of clinical trials that there activity in blocking HMG Co-A reductase activity inducing the LDL receptor thereby promoting the clearance of LDL from the circulation for ultimate secretion as bile acids. This has led to a striking decrease in all atherosclerotic affects, including myocardial infarction, angina, stroke, transient ischaemic attacks, peripheral vascular disease and vascular dementia. Overall, a 30% reduction has been demonstrated. Yet, a surprisingly large number of people of the order of 70% still go on to get events!

The development of mouse models through transgenesis and knockout by homologous recombination has revolutionised the study of atherosclerosis (Table 2; after Glass and Witztum, 2001). The apoE knockout mouse and the LDL receptor knockout mouse get human-like atherosclerotic lesions. On this background a large number of other molecules have been tested by transgenesis or knockout and been implicated in the development of atherosclerosis or protection against it.

The most important and early ongoing event in the development of atherosclerosis is the oxidation of LDL (Fig. 2, Table 3 and 4). This predominantly takes place within the arterial intima where the damaged apoB and lipids in LDL become ligands for the uptake by monocyte macrophage and for induction of the formation of foam cells. LDL uptake is mediated by the induction of specific receptors such as the scavenger receptors SRA and SRB. At the early stage, macrophage accumulation leads to the formation of fatty streaks with the activation of the overlying endothelium and the expression of adhesion molecules such as VCAM-I, P-selectin, E-selectin, ICAM-1. Monocytes are attracted into the arterial intima by secretion of chemokines and cytokines such as M-CSF.

Table 2. Genes and atherosclerosis in hypercholesterolaemic mice

Gene	Experiment	Genetic background	Effects on lesion area	Proposed mechanism
Atherogenic genes				
12/15-LO	KO	$apoE^{-/-}$	↓↓	Decreased LDL oxidation
	Overexpression	LDL $R^{-/-}$	↑	Increased LDL oxidation
iNOS	KO	$apoE^{-/-}$	↓	Decreased LDL oxidation
M-CSF	KO	$apoE^{-/-}$	↓↓	Decreased macrophage infiltration
MCP-1	KO	LDL $R^{-/-}$	↓↓	Decreased macrophage infiltration
		$apoE^{-/-}$		
CCR2	KO	$apoE^{-/-}$	↓↓	Decreased macrophage infiltration
P- and E-selectin	Combined KO	LDL $R^{-/-}$	↓	Decreased monocyte adherence
CXCR-2	KO	LDL $R^{-/-}$	↓	Decreased macrophage residence
SR-A	KO	$apoE^{-/-}$	↓	Decreased uptake of oxLDL
CD36	KO	$apoE^{-/-}$	↓↓	Decreased uptake of oxLDL
IFNγ receptor (R0)	KO	$apoE^{-/-}$	↓	Decreased inflammatory responses, increased apoAIV
CD154	KO	$apoE^{-/-}$	↓	Decreased CD40 signalling
IL-10	KO	C57 BL/6J	↑	Increased inflammatory response
Antiatherogenic genes				
Paraoxinase	KO	$apoE^{-/-}$	↑	Reduced clearance of oxidised lipids
apoA-1	KO	h apoB transgene	↑	Decreased reverse cholesterol transport
	Overexpression	$apoE^{-/-}$	↓	Increased reverse cholesterol transport
		LDL $R^{-/-}$		
PPARγ	KO	LDL $R^{-/-}$	↑	Altered macrophage function
	Agonist	LDL $R^{-/-}$	↓	
SR	KO	LDL $R^{-/-}$	↑	Decreased reverse cholesterol transport
	Overexpression	LDL $R^{-/-}$	↓	Increased reverse cholesterol transport

Table 3. Mechanisms of LDL oxidation

— 12/15-Lipoxygenase
— NAD(P)H oxidases
— Inflammatory PAF-like phospholipids
— Phospholipid oxidation products
— Oxidative DNA damage
— High-density lipoproteins in oxidation and inflammation
— NO positive and negative effects

Many mechanisms are now recognised for the production of oxidative damage to LDL through free radical production (Table 3 and 4; after Glass and Witztum, 2001). With animal studies, anti-oxidants have been moderately successful in preventing experimental atherosclerosis. Yet, in human studies, anti-oxidants, such as Vitamin E have been much less clearly successful (Glass and Witztum, 2001).

The cells of the atherosclerotic plaque

Intracellular interactions

The formation of the atherosclerotic plaque is brought about by a complex of cellular and molecular interactions (Fig. 1, 2 and 4). Substances expressed on

Table 4. Proatherogenic effects of ox LDL

oxLDL components	Effect	Mechanism
Lyso phosphatidyl choline (PC), oxidized phospholipids	Increased monocyte and T cell adhesion and recruitment	Increased expression of adhesion molecules on endothelial cells, chemokines like MLP-1, and G2A receptor
	Increased scavenger receptor A	Activate AP-1 and ets
9-hydroxyeicosatetraenoic acid	Increase CD36	Activation of PPARγ
	Induction of preinflammatory genes	Activation of NFκB, AP-1, and cAMP
Oxidized apoB and phospholipids	Increased foam cell formation	Enhanced uptake by scavenger receptor
Oxidized lipids and apoB adducts	Induces T and B cell responses	Neoepitope formation
Lyso PC, cholesterol, oxysterols	Increased apoptosis and necrosis	Cell death, formation of cholesterol crystals. Membrane damage
Oxidized lipids	Enhanced procoagulant activity	Induction of tissue factor and platelet aggregation

the surface and secreted in response to cellular activation bring about these events. Growth factors generally promote mitosis or cellular lymph plasma but can, in certain contexts, block cell growth or cause apoptosis. Cytokines because of their production from inflammatory cells and role in the generation of the inflammatory response. Many cytokines also act as growth factors and chemoattractants, and can inhibit cellular processes. Chemoattractants cause the movement of cells down a chemical gradient. Growth factors such as platelet-derived growth factor (PDGF) can also act as chemoattractants. Many of these substances are controlled by transcription factors, such as (NFKB), that respond to inflammation and have promoter elements that respond to sheer stress, for which transcription factors exist. Molecular interactions are often both autocrine and paracrine effects (Fig. 4).

Endothelial cells

In the earliest stage of atherogenesis, damaged endothelial cells become dysfunction (non-denuding injury). Sloughing of the endothelium occurs at a later stage in the disease, when plaques become complicated and split or fissure (denuding injury). The dysfunctional endothelial cells produces growth factors, cytokines, chemoattractants, clotting factors, and adhesion molecules. The result is the recruitment and transformation of monocytes into macrophages and the recruitment and transformation of smooth muscle cells. Thrombotic processes are activated at the endothelial cell surface. There is chronic alteration of vascular tone as a result of disordered NO production and signalling.

Monocyte/macrophages

The lipid-laden macrophage is the hallmark of atherosclerosis and the instrument of its development. The process of the monocyte conversion from a quiescent cell to the phagocytically active macrophage is associated with the expression of the scavenger receptor. The uptake of oxidatively modified LDL thus accompanies macrophage activation. The macrophage scavenger receptor is expressed in two differentially spliced forms. Both forms contain a collagen-like domain that binds polyanonic ligands, such as modified LDL. In modified LDL apoB loses its overall basic charge due to oxidation of critical lysine resides, such as those that mediate binding to acidic residues on the LDL receptor, and becomes covalently associated with lipid peroxidation products including short-chain aldehydes and ketones. This material is no longer taken up by the LDL receptor, but is avidly taken up by the macrophage scavenger receptor. The cholesteryl ester released from LDL is broken down in lysosomes and re-esterified in the cytoplasm.

The activated macrophage secretes a wide variety of growth-modulating substances and chemoattractants. Phagocytic macrophages produce free radicals and are induced to produce NO; this itself generates free radicals and promotes further oxidative damage to LDL. Macrophages also secrete proteolytic enzymes (collagenase, elastase, stromolysin and gelatinises). Proteases contribute to the necrosis and liquefaction of the core of advanced fatty plaques and render the plaque prone to rupture, either into the arterial lumen or through the external wall it the form of aneurismal rupture.

Vascular smooth muscle cells

In the normal artery wall smooth muscle cells contain mainly contractile proteins, such as actin and myosin. These cells are said to display a contractile phenotype. They respond to vasoregulatory substances such as catecholamines, angiotensis II, prostaglandins, leukotrienes, endothelin, NO, and other regulatory compounds. Under the influence of pro-inflammatory cytokines and growth factors, smooth muscle cells in the atherosclerotic plaque switch from a contractile to a secretory phenotype. These cells have large amounts

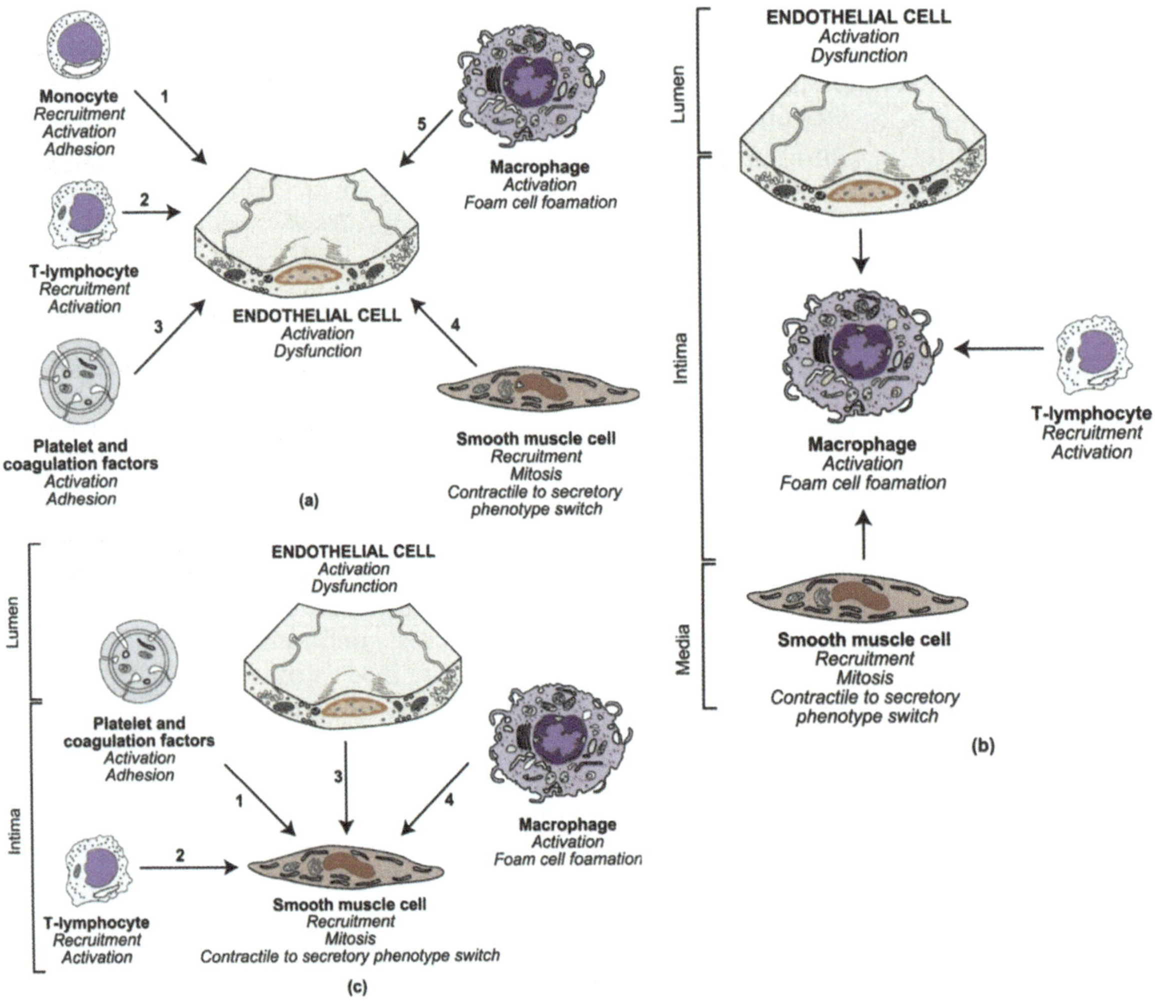

of endoplasmic reticulum and Golgi apparatus. They produce matrix proteins. The local release of froth factors, cytokines, and chemoattractants leads to autocrine and paracrine effects on growth and cell recruitment. Smooth muscle cells also express a scavenger receptor and they, took become lipid loaded.

Lymphocytes

Both B and T lymphocyte accompany macrophages into the atherosclerotic plaque. They too produce proinflammatory cytokines which compound the atherosclerotic process by attracting further macrophages. They also perpetuate endothelial cell activation through cytokine production.

Platelets

Platelets undergo activation in response to agonists such as thrombin, ADP adrenaline, and plately activating factor. This process is also triggered when

Fig. 4. Cellular and molecular mediators of atherosclerosis. The arrows denote the production of factors and their principal cellular targets. **a** Endothelial cells Monocytes are recruited and adhere to the vascular endothelium, where extravasation and activation occurs. In the process of activation the monocyte is transformed into the phagocytically active macrophage and produces numerous growth factors, growth inhibitors, and chemoattractants. (ii) T-lymphocytes undergo recruitment and activation. They secrete γ-interferon (IFNγ), transforming growth factor β(TGFβ), tumour necrosis factor α (TNFα), and interleukin-1 (IL-1). (iii) platelet activation and adhesion is associated with coagulation cascade activation. Platelet degranulation and prostaglandin production occurs with release of platelet derived growth factor(PDGF) epidermal growth factor (EFG)/TGFα, TGFβ, thromboxane A and insulin-like growth factor I (IFG-1). (iv) Smooth muscle cells switch to a secretory phenotype and produce vascular endothelial cell growth factor (VEFG), IL-1, TNFα, TGFβ, collagen, elastic fibres, and proteoglycans. (v) Macrophages become phagocytically active. The scavenger receptor is induced with the engorgement of oxidized low-density lipoprotein (oxLDL) and foam cell formation. Activated macrophages produced VEGF, IL-1, TNFα, IFNγ. **b** Macrophage; (i) Endothelial cells become activated and dysfunctional. They secrete macrophage colony stimulating factor (M-CSF)/granulocyte-macrophage colony-stimulating factor (GM-CSF), IL-1, TNFα, macrophage chemotactic protein 1 (MCP-1) and take up oxLDL. (ii) Smooth muscle cells are recruited and my divide before switching from a contractile to a secretory phenotype. They secrete M-CSF/GM-CSF, heparin-binding epidermal growth factor (HB-EGF), VEGF, IL-1, TNFα, MCP-1, and produce oxLDL. (iii) T cells are recruited and secrete IFNγ, GM-CSF TNFα. Macrophage IL-2 is a potent agent for T-cell recruitment and activation. **c** Smooth muscle cells; (i) Platelets are activated and produce PDGF, EGF/TGFα, TGFβ, TXA_2 and IGF-1. (ii) T lymphocytes become activated and produced (TFNγ), TGFβ, TNFα, and IL-1. (iii) Endothelial cells produce PDGF, basic fibroblast growth factor (bFGF), IL-1, TGFβ, prostaglandin I_2 (PGI_2), IGF-1, nitric oxide (NO), and oxLDL. (iv) Macrophage produce PDGF, bFGF, HB-EFF, TGFα, TGFβ, TNFα, IL-1, prostaglandin E (PGE), and ox LDL (based on Ross, 1999; Scott, 1995; Naoumova and Scott, 2000; Glass and Witzum, 2001; Libby, 2001)

peripheral blood is exposed to thrombogenic agents at the site of blood vessel damage. Here agonists such as collagen present in the extracellular matrix, exposed to the subendothelium along with von Willebrand factor and fibrinogen produced at the wound site, initiate the cascade of events that leads to platelet aggregation and the formation of a platelet plug. In this process platelet-specific integrins act as receptor tyrosine kinases (GPIIbIIIa), which initiative the intracellular changes that mediate platelet activation and aggregation, and later binding to fibrin and clot.

The unstable plaque

With time, the mature plaque becomes unstable (Fig. 2). The process of becoming unstable and vulnerable to rupture is mediated by the dynamic events going on in the plaque. Macrophage proteases liquefy the core of the plaque. Smooth muscle cells undergo apoptosis. The corners and surface of plaques become thin and prone to rupture. Tissue factor is expressed in the macrophage so that should rupture occur there is the potential for explosive and devastating thrombosis. Often a more subtle modulated process of platelet embolisation leads to transient ischaemic attacks or other vascular events elsewhere. Statin drugs have a key role in stabilising the plaque against rupture (Table 5; after Libby, 2001).

Beyond statin treatment

Although reduction of circulating LDL cholesterol levels with statins has had a major impact of the burden of atherosclerosis, many (70%) of people still go on to have events. Perhaps intervention has been too late, and the disease too progressed to prevent lesion rupture and the manifestations of disease. A key advance would be to develop surrogates of advancing disease so that the question could be answered as to whether this young man or woman has advanced disease in early life and therefore must undergo aggressive intervention in order to prevent later life events.

Table 5. Beneficial effects of lipid lowering

Reduces	Increases
Macrophage number	Interstitial collagen content
Matrix metalloproteinase expression	Smooth muscle maturation
Tissue factor gene expression	
Proinflammatory cytokine expression	
Leukocyte adhesion molecule expression	
Production of reactive oxygen species	

Table 6. Markers, surrogates and measures of atherosclerotic risk

- Circulatory surrogates
  - — C reactive protein
  - — Serum amyloid A
  - — Intercellular adhesion molecule-I
  - — Soluble E-selectin
  - — Matrix metalloproteinases
  - — Solube CD40 ligand
  - — NMR of plasma
- Imaging
  - — CMRI, ultrasound, ECHO, ultrafast (EB) CT, PET, SPECT

Surrogates for atherosclerosis are now available (Table 6; after Libby, 2001). Perhaps the best of these is C reactive protein. Others include serum amyloid A, intracellular adhesion molecule 1, soluble E-selectin, circulating matrix metaloproteinases, soluble CD40 ligand. In addition, a number of new imaging modalities including NMR, ultrasound, CT and PET, may have a role in predicting early disease and indicating the need for early intervention. Despite a plethora of key molecules (Figure legend 4 and Table 7; after Glass and Witztum, 2001) that might be used as potential interventions in preventing plaque progression, the identification and validation of targets is a long,

Table 7. Potential targets of inhibitors of atherosclerosis

Target	Drug	Mechanism of action
15-lipoxygenase	Inhibitor	Inhibition of LDL oxidation in arterial wall
MTP	Inhibitor	Inhibition of VLDL secretion from liver
CCR2	Antagonist	Inhibition of monocyte recruitment to vessel wall
Endothelin A receptor	Antagonist	Inhibition of hypoxic vasoconstriction
MMPs	Inhibitor	Prevention of plaque rupture
CETP	Inhibitor	Increased HDL and reverse cholesterol transport
ABC1	Agonist	Increase cholesterol efflux and HDC
Potential transcription factor inhibitors of atherosclerosis		
1κB kinase	Inhibitor	Inhibition of NFκB decreases inflammation
PPARα	Agonist	Decreased TG-rich lipoproteins, increased HDL, anti-inflammatory
PPARγ	Selective modulator	Decreased insulin resistance and anti-inflammatory in macrophages
LXRα	Selective modulator	Decreased cholesterol absorption, increased hepatic excretion and increased efflux cholesterol from macrophages
RXR	Selective modulator	Activation of PPAR and LXR pathways (induce hypertriglyceridaemia and hypothyroidism)
ERα,β	Selective modulator	Improved lipoprotein profiles and arterial wall biology

laborious process. The development of drugs that ultimately do not work well or are toxic has serious financial consequences for the pharmaceutical industry.

Some old approaches and some new approaches

In addition to the advances coming from the use of transgenic and knockout mice models, traditional linkage studies in Mendelian disorders have yielded a rich harvest. The microsomal triglyceride transfer protein MTP was identified as a key molecule for the loading of apoB with triglyceride within the cell (Natcisi et al., 1993). As such, MTP inhibitors became key targets for drug discovery and compounds were developed across the pharmaceutical industry. Unfortunately, through mechanism of action, the failure to secrete triglyceride from the cell, a serious mechanism of action based complication was massive fatty liver. In addition, the compounds were not better than the statins. Thus, despite being an interesting tool for the investigation of the detailed mechanisms of secretion of apoB they have not found favour as new drugs for the treatment of disease.

Much more promising has been the discovery of the molecular defect in Tangier disease (Fig. 5) (Scott, 1999). Tangier disease named after a family with the disorder on Tangier Island in Chesapeake Bay is a disorder in which no normal HDL is formed. As a consequence, subjects get lipid engorged macrophages in the tonsils, spleen, and indeed, in some subjects, in the arterial wall. It was discovered by several groups that a gene on chromosome 9 responsible for the efflux of cholesterol and phospholipid from the cell was defective in this disorder. This gene encodes a protein ABCA1 belonging to a large family of proteins involved in the movement of substances across the cellular membrane. In the early states of atherogenesis ABCA1 transports the cholesterol from the cell for uptake by nascent HDL lipoproteins containing mainly apoA1 and phospholipids. Thus, ABCA1 which is regulated at the level of transcription, phosphorylation, through its requirement for ATP and as on ion channel seems to be an ideal target for drug discovery. Indeed, now, studies with transgenic mice that over express ABCA1 indicate that this may be the case. A recent crystal structure for a member of the ABC transporter family may help in the molecular design of such potential compounds.

Thus far, the use of linkage studies to identify the causes of complex disease have yielded a much less rich harvest. Linkage is a relatively blunt instrument and has only to date identified genes causal of diabetes mellitus and Crohns disease despite a huge International effort. Nonetheless, there is still a large repertoire of potential drugs, therapeutic targets. Some of these are involved in oxidative free radical production (Table 7). Those are transcription factors that have key roles in atherogenesis. Already some of these are drug ligands that modulate their activity such as PPARα and PPARγ.

The power of the now available sequence of the human genome has begun to yield its rich harvest. Transcriptomics and proteomics are yielding a new harvest of molecules, active in the risk cascades for atherogenesis and within

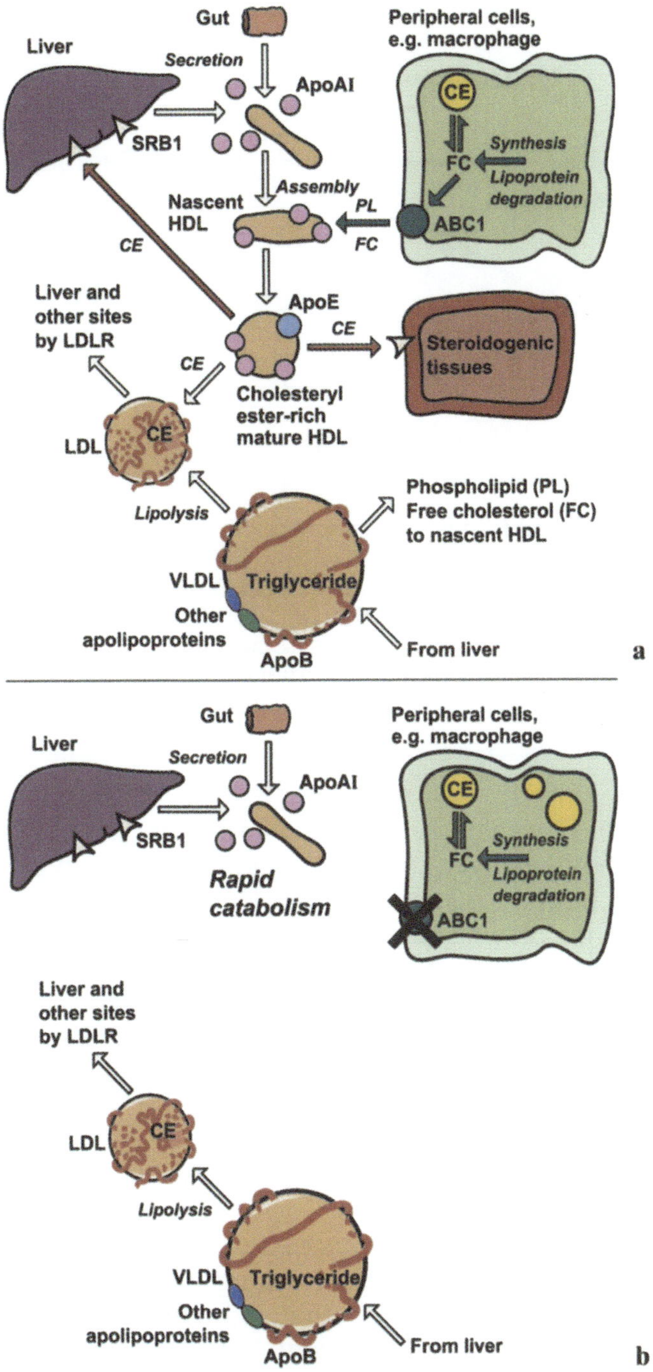

Fig. 5. Cholesterol and Tangier disease. **a** The Newly discovered cholesterol-efflux regulatory protein is necessary for the bulk transfer of free cholesterol (FC)mand phospholipid (PL) out of cells. In the extracellular fluid, apolipoprotein-AI (apoAI) and nascent high-density lipoprotein (HDL) act as acceptors for the cholesterol. The free cholesterol in mature HDL is esterified (cholesteryl ester, CE) and transferred to low-density lipoprotein (LDL) and to cells by scavenger receptor B1 (SRB1). ApoB is the main apolipoprotein in LDL and very low-density lipoprotein (VLDL). So, in normal cells, ApoAI is recycled. **b** In patients with Tangier disease, however, the absence of free cholesterol and phospholipid aborts the formation of HDL owing to defects. The apoAI is rapidly cleared from the circulation and degraded. Events that are effective in Tangier disease are shaded

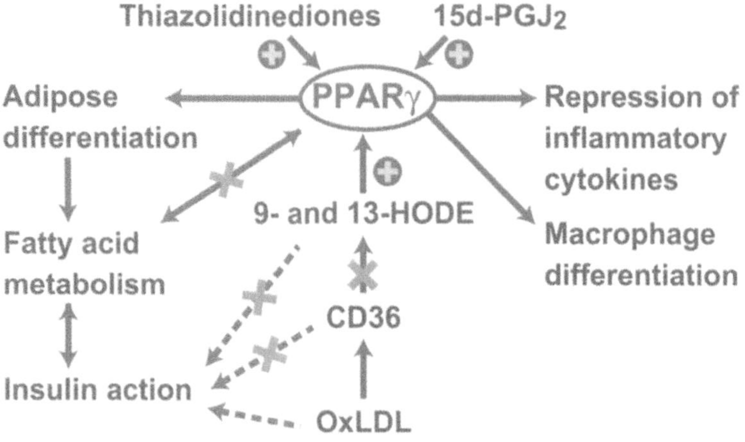

Fig. 6. Role of CD36 and PPARγ in insulin action and atherogenesis. Activated PPARγ induces transcription of CD36. CD36 takes up 9-HODE and 13-HODE, the linoleic acid components of oxidised LDL, which activate PPARγ, further increasing transcription of CD36. The mechanisms by which PPARγ and CD36 affect insulin action, and the extent of overlap between the two pathways, remain unclear. *15d-PGJ2* 15-deoxy-Δ12,14-prostaglandin J_2, *HODE* Hydroxyoctadecadienoic acid, *X* blocked in CD36 deficiency

the arterial wall. For example, in our own hands, we were able to combine conventional Mendelian genetics in the spontaneously hypertensive rat — an animal that gets insulin resistance, dyslipidaemia and hypertension, to identify a single gene with a pleotropic effect on all of these phenotypes. Surprisingly, this gene is a fatty acid transporter called CD36 and is one of the macrophage scavenger receptors (Fig. 6) (Aitman et al., 1999; Aitman, 2001). It is highly regulated by PPARγ and as such its induction may have a key role in insulin sensitisation.

Concluding remarks

It can be anticipated that the pharmaceutical sector working with medical and non-medical scientists will develop new drugs that will have a key role in the prevention of atherosclerosis. Nonetheless, many of the risk factors causing disease are already known and preventable. You only have to observe the catalogue (Table 1) of risk factors known for this disorder to realise that simple interventions can prevent disease. A major, major issue in prevention is, however, going to be compliance. How do we prevent and treat obesity? How do we stop people smoking? How do we encourage a more healthy lifestyle? In the words of Macbeth (Act III, Scene II) after he killed his key rival Banquo, while fortunately Banquo's son Fleance escaped, cursed "We have scotch'd the snake, not kill'd it." This is the situation with atherosclerosis today. There have been huge advances, but there is a huge distance to travel.

References

Aitman TJ (2001) CD36, insulin resistance and coronary heart disease. Lancet 357: 651–652

Aitman T, Glazier A, Wallace C, Cooper L, Norsworthy O, Wahid F, Al-Majali K, Trembling P, Mann C, Shoulders C, Graf D, S.Lezin E, Kurtz T, Kren V, Pravenec M, Ibrahimi A, Abumrad N, Stanton L, Scott J (1999) Identification of CD36I (Fat) as an insulin-resistance gene causing defective fatty acid and glucose metabolism in hyperactive rats. Nature Genet 21: 76–83

Glass CK, Witztum JL (2001) Atherosclerosis: the road ahead. Cell 104: 503–516

Libby P (2001) Current concepts of the pathogenesis of the acute coronary syndromes. Circulation 104: 365

Narcisi YM, Scholtz MC, Scott J, Shoulders CC (1993) Dinucleotide repeat polymorphisms at the lipoprotein lipase (LPL) locus. Hum Genet 92: 312–313

Naumova RP, Scott J (2000) The pathogenesis of atherosclerosis. In: Weatherall DJ, Ledingham JGE, Warrell DA (eds) Concise Oxford Textbook of Medicine. Oxford University Press, pp 48–50

Ross R (1999) Atherosclerosis — an inflammatory disease. N Engl J Med 340: 115–125

Scott J (1995) The pathogenesis of atherosclerosis. Oxford Book of Medicine 2: 2289–2295

Scott J (1999) Good cholesterol news. Nature 400: 816–819

Stamler J, Wentworth D, Neaton JD (1986) Is relationship between serum cholesterol and risk of premature death from coronary heart disease continuous and graded? Findings in 356,222 primary screenees of the Multiple Risk Factor Intervention Trial (MRFIT). JAMA 256(20): 2823–2828

Author's address: Prof. J. Scott, FRS, Imperial College Genetics and Genomics Research Institute, National Heart & Lung Institute, Faculty of Medicine, Imperial College of Science, Technology and Medicine, Hammersmith Campus, Du Cane Road, London W12 ONN, United Kingdom, e-mail: j.scott@ic.ac.uk

J Neural Transm (2002) [Suppl] 63: 19–36

Stroke: imaging and differential diagnosis

J. C. Baron

Department of Neurology and Stroke Unit, University of Cambridge, United Kingdom

Summary. Structural and vascular imaging helps to differentiate haemorrhagic from acute ischemic stroke (AIS) and rule out non-stroke causes, as well as identify specific subtypes of stroke such as carotid dissection and venous thrombosis. However, it is negative in most AIS patients within 3–6 hrs of onset and thus does not allow efficient patient classification for management purposes. Physiologic neuroimaging with PET, SPECT and combined diffusion- and perfusion-weighted MR gives access to tissue perfusion and cell function/homeostasis. It has near 100% sensitivity in AIS, even in small cortical or brainstem strokes. In middle-cerebral artery (MCA) stroke, physiologic imaging also allows pathophysiological differentiation into four tissue subtypes: i) already irreversibly damaged ("core"); ii) severely hypoperfused ("penumbra"), which represents the main target for therapy; iii) mildly hypoperfused ("oligaemia"), not at risk of infarction unless secondary complications arise; and iv) reperfused/hyperperfused. PET studies have evidenced the penumbra in man, shown its largely cortical topography, documented its anticipated impact on both acute-stage neurological deficit and recovery therefrom, and shown its persistence up to 16 hrs after stroke onset in some patients. However, some patients acutely exhibit extensive irreversible damage, which places them at considerable risk of malignant MCA infarction, and others early spontaneous reperfusion, which is almost invariably associated with rapid and complete recovery. Thrombolytics and/or neuroprotective agents would therefore be expected to benefit, and hence should ideally be reserved to, only those patients in whom a substantial penumbra is documented by physiologic neuroimaging, even perhaps beyond the 3 to 6 hrs rule. In addition, excluding from thrombolytic therapy those patients with substantial necrotic core should avoid many instances of symptomatic haemorrhagic transformations. Finally, patients with extensive core might benefit from early decompressive surgery, and those with early extensive reperfusion from anti-inflammatory agents. Overall, therefore, the pathophysiologic heterogeneity underlying AIS may account for both the complications from thrombolysis and the limited success of clinical trials of neuroprotective agents, despite apparent benefit in the laboratory. Pathophysiological diagnosis as afforded by neuroimaging should now be incorporated in the design of clinical trials as well as in the routine management of stroke.

Introduction

Imaging has revolutionized the approach to acute MCA territory stroke (operationally defined here as the first 24 hours after onset of clinical symptoms). Introduced in the 50s, classic *angiography* allows the visualization of the neck and brain vessels and therefore shows the occluded vessel (carotid or vertebro-basilar and their branches) but can be normal if the artery occluded is too small or if the clot has dissolved spontaneously or as a result of therapy. Angiography may also detect a potential proximal source of emboli, e.g. a stenosis of the origin of the internal carotid artery in the neck. A more considerable revolution took place with the advent of *structural brain imaging*, first with X-ray CT scanning in the 70s, and MRI in the 80s. These techniques allow the identification of tissue damage, i.e., infarcts (large or lacunar), white matter ischemic changes, subarachnoid or parenchymal haemorrhage, and microbleeds. In addition, both CT and MR allow to visualize clots within blood vessels or in the artery wall (dissection) and to obtain angiography with a resolution getting closer to that of formal arteriograms with technique improvements (see Fig. 2 for an illustration). Finally, *functional neuroimaging* uniquely provides maps of brain physiology such as tissue perfusion and metabolism. Imaging of these variables in stroke not only has permitted major pathophysiologic insights into the understanding of acute cerebral ischemia, but also is now considered of major importance in clinical trials and patient management since it allows patient classification according to pathophysiology rather than clinical and structural imaging data only. The main functional neuroimaging techniques are positron emission tomography (PET), which is considered gold standard because it provides quantitative mapping of many physiologic parameters but is complex, costly and not readily available, and a number of more clinically accessible techniques such as single photon emission tomography (SPECT), stable Xenon CT (Xe-CT), and MR-based diffusion-weighted and perfusion imaging. Another application of MR is spectroscopy to quantitate local concentrations of tissue biochemicals and neurotransmitters. The focus in this paper will be on functional neuroimaging, but the reader interested in an overview of structural and angiographic techniques as applied to stroke is referred to textbooks and specific reviews (Ginsberg and Bogousslavsky, 1998; Heiss et al., 2001).

Brief overview of techniques

A detailed overview of the methods used in functional neuroimaging can be found ealsewhere (Baron et al., 1989; Baron and Marchal, 2000), so only a brief summary will be given here. Regarding *PET*, several approaches are possible. Using ^{15}O labeled tracers such as H_2O, CO_2, CO, and O_2, and the glucose analogue ^{18}F-fluoro-2-deoxy-D-glucose (FDG), quantitative mapping of the cerebral blood flow (CBF), cerebral blood volume (CBV), cerebral metabolic rate of oxygen ($CMRO_2$), oxygen extraction fraction (OEF), and brain glucose utilization (CMRGlc) can be obtained. The use of ^{18}FDG to measure CMRglc in acute stroke may be complicated by unpredictable changes in the "lumped constant". Access to CBF and CBV allows computing the CBV/CBF ratio, which represents the mean transit time (MTT), while the reverse ratio CBF/CBV is an index of the local cerebral perfusion pressure (CPP). PET can also be used to measure intracellular pH (Syrota et al., 1985; Senda et al., 1985). Of interest for cerebrovascular disease are also three specific markers: i) ^{11}C-flumazenil (^{11}C-FMZ), a benzodiazepine receptor radioligand (Sette et al., 1993) which is used as a marker of neuronal integrity; ii) ^{11}C-PK 11-195 (^{11}C-PK), a peripheral benzodiazepine radioligand which reflects glial inflammation (Ramsay et al., 1992; Sette et al., 1993); and iii) ^{18}F-fluoro-misonidazole (^{18}F-MISO), a marker of tissue hypoxia (Read et al., 1998).

Xe-CT allows the mapping of CBF, with however limitations due to constraints on the number of brain cuts that can be obtained, small signal-to-noise ratio, and behavioural effects of cold xenon. *SPECT* with ^{99m}Tc-HMPAO allows the mapping of tissue perfusion but quantitation is difficult, and the tracer's behaviour can deviate from perfusion in a number of pathophysiological situations. ^{99m}Tc-ECD brain uptake is determined by both perfusion and cell homeostasis, an interesting feature for pathophysiological investigations but which may raise issues about interpretation of the findings in the clinical setting. SPECT benzodiazepine radioligands have also been developed for use in clinical research.

Regarding *MR*, diffusion-weighted imaging (DWI) assesses the compartmentation of water in brain tissue. From the DWI images the apparent diffusion coefficient of water (ADC) can be calculated. Within minutes of onset of cerebral ischemia, mapping of ADC documents reduced water diffusion, reflecting cytotoxic edema and thus failure of cell energy status (Baird and Warach, 1998). Using T2* imaging, perfusion-weighted gadolinium bolus tracking derives semi-quantitative maps of MTT, CBV and CBF from the time course of the tracer; absolute quantification of perfusion parameters is however still restricted. MR spectroscopy (MRS) assesses important cellular biochemicals such as N-acetyl-aspartate (NAA, a specific neuronal marker) and lactate with proton MRS. Most applications so far have been with single-volume MRS, but imaging with acceptable resolution is feasible, especially with high-field new generation magnets (Gillard et al., 1996; Kamada et al., 1997).

Findings with PET

PET permits to operationally characterize the individual pathophysiological situation in acute ischemic stroke. Brain tissue can be classified into four subtypes: i) the core (defined as the irreversibly damaged tissue already present at time of imaging); ii) the penumbra (defined as that severely hypoperfused tissue at risk of, but that can still be saved from, infarction); iii) the oligemia (defined as mildly hypoperfused and not at-risk of infarction under normal circumstances); and iv) the hyperperfused tissue (defined as that tissue with CBF higher than that in the contralateral homologous tissue, and taken to represent effective reperfusion).

Mapping the core

Methods: Mapping the core depicts the extent of that tissue which is already beyond therapeutic reach and potentially at risk of hemorrhagic transformation especially with the use of thrombolytics. A $CMRO_2$ threshold about 0.9 ml/100 ml.min has been validated for voxel-based studies done in the 5–18 hrs interval (Marchal et al., 1999). The corresponding threshold for CBF is ~8.5 mls/100 ml.min, but contrary to oxygen consumption, the CBF threshold is expected to depend on time since occlusion. Accordingly, a CBF infarction threshold around 5 mls/100 g.min has recently been reported from studies performed within 6 hrs of stroke studies (Heiss et al., 2001). Heiss et al. (2001) also recently computed a cortical irreversibility threshold for ^{11}C-Flumazenil within 12 hrs of stroke onset, as less than 3.4 times the white matter value.

Findings: In many patients, and consistent with its end-artery vascular system, the striato-capsular area very early exhibits irreversible damage, in striking contrast with the cortical mantle which demonstrates penumbra (see below and Fig. 1) (Wise et al., 1983; Marchal et al., 1993). In some patients, however, the core may widely extend into cortical areas as early as 4–6 hours after stroke onset (Marchal et al., 1993, 1995), suggesting inadequate pial collaterals or proximal carotid occlusion in these people (Fig. 1). The volume of core is highly linearly correlated to both the severity of admission neurological deficit and final infarct volume, as assessed by structural imaging in the chronic stage (Marchal et al., 1999). However, core volume underestimated the latter by a factor of two, because of subsequent metabolic deterioration of

Fig. 1. Illustrative PET patterns in acute MCA territory stroke. This figure illustrates the three PET patterns of CBF and $CMRO_2$ changes observed within 18 hrs of onset of MCA territory stroke. The *top row* shows an example of *early extensive irreversible damage* in a patient with right-sided MCA territory stroke studied with PET 17 hours after symptom onset. There was a near zero CBF and $CMRO_2$ in the whole right MCA territory, together with patchy OEF (black pixels represent unmeasurable OEF). *Penumbra* (*middle row*): in this patient with acute-stage right MCA territory stroke, the PET study performed 12 hours after onset revealed a markedly reduced CBF in the whole right MCA territory, associated with relatively preserved $CMRO_2$ (except in the lenticulo-striate area) and extremely elevated OEF (misery perfusion). The *bottom row* images illustrate an example of *early luxury perfusion* in a patient studied with PET 13 hours after onset of right-sided MCA territory stroke. There is markedly increased CBF in the central right MCA territory, associated with normal or slightly increased $CMRO_2$ and decreased OEF

Fig. 2. Mismatch with DWI-PWI MR. This figure illustrates a typical "mismatch" between extensive reduction in perfusion in the entire left carotid territory but DWI abnormality restricted to the lenticulo-capsulo-caudate area in a patient studied 4 hrs after clinical onset of left hemiparesis. Note that MR angiography shows occluded right internal carotid artery intracranially, due to dissection in this patient

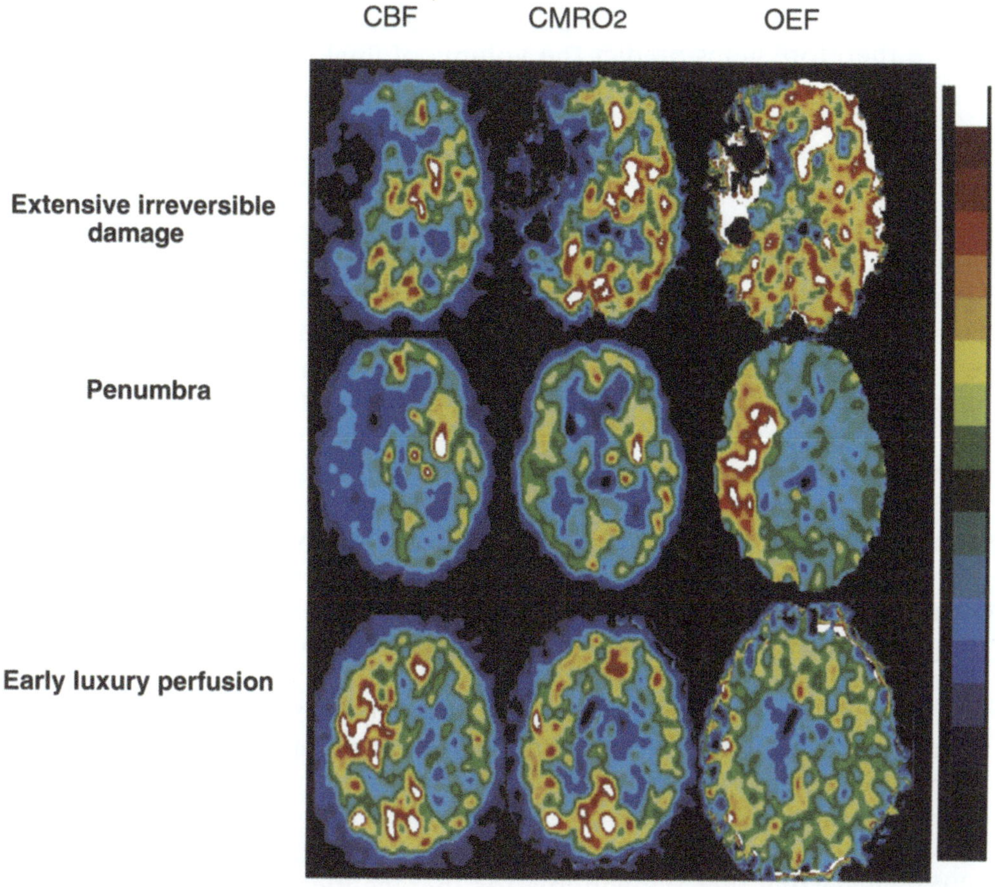
CBF
CMRO2
OEF
Extensive irreversible damage
Penumbra
Early luxury perfusion

Fig. 1

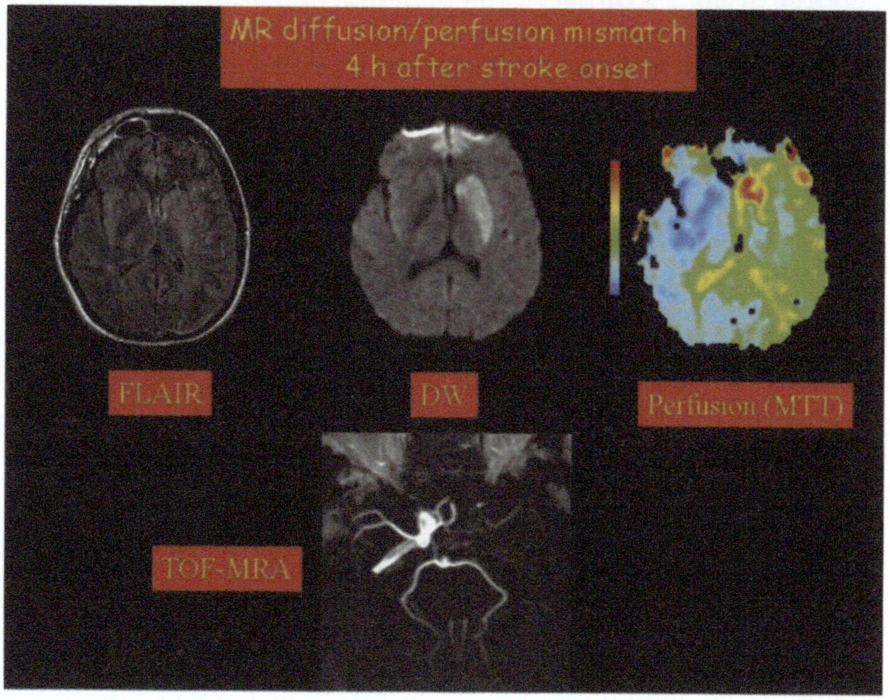
MR diffusion/perfusion mismatch
4 h after stroke onset
FLAIR
DW
Perfusion (MTT)
TOF-MRA

Fig. 2

the penumbra (see below). Mapping the ischemic core in the acute stage of stroke therefore helps predict the volume of final infarction.

Mapping the penumbra

Methods: as already stated, acute-stroke PET often demonstrates critical ischemia affecting wide zones of the cortex and with features consistent with penumbra (Baron et al., 1981; Wise et al., 1983; Marchal et al., 1993) (Fig. 1). This tissue displays severe "misery perfusion" (Baron et al., 1981), that is, severely reduced CBF (i.e., below the penumbral threshold of ~20 ml/100 ml/minute), strikingly increased OEF (often above 0.8 for a normal of about 0.4), and relatively preserved $CMRO_2$ (i.e., above the threshold for viability defined above). Furlan et al. (1996) reported a range of CBF characterizing this tissue of 7–17 mls/100 ml.min, close to the penumbra range reported in monkeys (Astrup et al., 1981; Jones et al., 1981). Marchal et al. (1996) also found a penumbra threshold of 22 mls/100 g.min close to classic experimental data. Heiss et al. (2001) recently reported a penumbra threshold of 14.5 mls/100 g.min, which lies on the low side presumably for methodological reasons (Baron, 2001).

Findings: both the incidence and the extent of penumbra tend to decrease with elapsing time since stroke onset. Substantial cortical penumbra has been reported in 90% of patients studied within 6 hrs from onset, in over 50% of the patients studied within 9 hours, and in about one third of patients studied between 5 and 18 hrs (Heiss et al., 1998, 2001; Wise et al., 1983; Marchal et al., 1995), suggesting that the window for therapeutic opportunity may be protracted in at least a subset of the patients. In one study, it was found that up to 52% (average: 32%) of the ultimately infarcted tissue still exhibited penumbra as late as 16 hrs after symptom onset (Marchal et al., 1996). Based on semi-quantitative data, Heiss et al. (1998) reported a smaller penumbral compartment (average: 18%) even though their patients were studied within 3 hrs of onset. However, they used an unconventional classification of tissue subtypes evolving to infarction which considered a mildly hypoperfused component as distinct from penumbra, despite being clearly at-risk of infarction. If this compartment is merged with their penumbra, then their findings would be consistent with the earlier reports. In a more recent report, Heiss et al. (2001) found a penumbra of about 20%, but again if the mildly hypoperfused compartment is included, then the at-risk compartment rises to 45% on average and up to 85% individually. Interestingly, in that study, large fractions of at-risk tissue were found 12 hrs from onset, confirming that in some patients with MCA territory stroke, a sizeable cortical penumbra may linger on for hours. Using ^{18}F-MISO, Read et al. (1998) reported that the volume of hypoxic brain tissue declined with elapsing time since stroke onset but was still substantial as late as 43 hrs; it must be recalled, however, that hypoxic tissue may represent simple oligemia.

Fate of the penumbra: the available PET data have demonstrated that the penumbra can either progress to or in part or in all escape infarction, depending on subsequent events such as reperfusion- either spontaneous or therapeutic (Baron, 1999). The demise of the penumbra is signalled by a decline in $CMRO_2$, while the CBF further declines or remains stable (Wise et al., 1983; Heiss et al., 1992; Marchal et al., 1996). This process is epitomized by a dramatic fall in the OEF, from initially very high to sometimes exceedingly low values (i.e., "luxury perfusion"), signalling the exhaustion of the tissue's oxygen needs. Studies in baboons have documented that early reperfusion is capable of reversing the otherwise deleterious fate of the penumbra (Touzani et al., 1995, 1997). In humans, Heiss et al. (1998) have reported that large volumes of tissue with penumbral levels of CBF escape necrosis in patients successfully recanalized by iv thrombolysis administered within 3 hrs from onset.

Mapping the oligemia

As stated above, the oligemic tissue is by definition hypoperfused but in principle not at risk of infarction. In other words, it displays a mild degree of misery perfusion with high OEF, but its CBF stands above the penumbra threshold. Furlan et al. (1996) documented that while in some patients the high OEF area was largely penumbral, in others it was virtually entirely oligemic. Thus, misery perfusion should not be equated with penumbra in acute stroke. As mentioned above, Heiss et al. (1999, 2001) found that, according to their tissue classification scheme, a substantial portion (≥45% in three patients) of the ultimate infarction was only mildly hypoperfused, i.e., oligemic. This observation serves to stress the point that, because its perfusion is pressure-dependent, the oligemic compartment, though not at risk of infarction in uncomplicated circumstances, may become incorporated in the penumbra, and hence potentially into the core, as a result of secondary events that tend to reduce the local CPP such as vasogenic oedema and systemic hypotension. It is also possible that cells in the oligemic tissue are sensitive to systemic factors that aggravate the flow-to-metabolism mismatch, such as hyperglycemia and pyrexia (Baron, 2001). These considerations are important because they would explain the benefits from avoiding such complications in the clinic.

Mapping hyperperfusion

Spontaneous hyperperfusion affecting the cortical mantle extensively or patchily, and sometimes the basal ganglia as well, has been observed in about one-third of the cases studied 5–18 hrs after stroke (Marchal et al., 1993, 1995) (Fig. 1). It is associated with reduced OEF and increased CBV, indicating luxury perfusion (Lassen, 1966; Baron et al., 1981; Ackerman et al., 1981) with abnormal vasodilatation. In most instances, the hyperperfused tissue exhibits mildly increased $CMRO_2$, suggesting post-ischemic rebound of cellular processes, and integrity at late structural imaging (Marchal et al., 1996), suggesting early hyperperfusion is a marker of good tissue prognosis. This pattern suggests that recanalization spontaneously occurred prior to PET and resulted in efficient reperfusion of the penumbra, consistent with the well-established notion that infarct size is reduced by early recanalization (Young et al., 1997). These observations in humans furthermore suggest that the experimental concept according to which sudden reoxygenation might exacerbate ischemic brain damage may not apply to man (see Marchal et al., 1999b, for review). However, hyperperfusion developing after therapeutic thrombolysis occasionally heralds poor tissue outcome (Heiss et al., 2000). One interpretation of this discrepancy with spontaneous recanalization is that thrombolysis may force reperfusion into an already irreversibly damaged vascular tree.

Pathophysiological heterogeneity and clinical correlates

In 30 patients investigated in the 5–18 hrs post-stroke interval, we prospectively assessed the relationships between acute-stage PET findings and clinical outcome (Marchal et al., 1993, 1995). There was considerable pathophysiological heterogeneity in this sample, unpredictable from neurological status. Thus, about one-third of the patients each could be classified into one of the three patterns of PET changes described above (Fig. 1), namely: i) extensive subcortico-cortical core (*Pattern 1*); ii) presence of penumbra without extensive core (*Pattern 2*; this pattern would equate with the "mismatch" pattern observed with diffusion-weighted and perfusion MR); and iii) hyperperfusion without extensive core (*Pattern 3*). There was a highly significant relationship between these patterns and subsequent neurological course. Thus, all pattern 1 patients did poorly (malignant infarction with early death or poor outcome), whereas all patients classified as pattern 3 did well (complete or nearly complete recovery in all). Consistent with the penumbra concept, pattern 2 patients had an unpredictable course, ranging from death to full recovery. Importantly, the PET patterns had significant independent predictive value for recovery over and above that of clinical scores alone (Marchal et al., 1995). Consistent findings have been reported by Heiss et al. (1997), who showed in a few cases studied both pre- and post- early iv thrombolysis that the occurrence of hyperperfusion was generally associated with good clinical and tissular outcome, unlike severe and persisting hypoperfusion.

Penumbra and neurological recovery

PET studies have documented that survival of the penumbra is one major determinant of recovery after ischaemic stroke. Furlan et al. (1996) found that the volume of penumbra that eventually escapes infarction had high correlation with the extent of subsequent neurological recovery. Likewise, Heiss et al. (1998) reported a significant correlation between the volume of critically hypoperfused tissue saved by thrombolysis and the change in neurological scores between admission and 3 weeks. Using ^{18}F-MISO, Read et al. (2000)

reported that the degree of neurological deterioration or improvement after MCA territory stroke was significantly related to the volume of initially hypoxic tissue that went on to infarct at subsequent structural imaging. Thus, all these data indicate that saving the penumbra has definite and predictable benefit on subsequent neurological recovery in man. Less predictably, the best correlation in Furlan et al's data was observed with 2-month recovery scores, suggesting that survival of the penumbra influences not only early, but also late, recovery, i.e., it provides an opportunity for subsequent peri-infarct neuronal reorganization.

Findings with SPECT and Xe-CT

Overall, SPECT with ^{99m}Tc-HMPAO and ^{99m}Tc-ECD in acute stroke has yielded findings consistent with PET, although with substantially lower accuracy due to lower spatial resolution, uncertain interpretation in terms of perfusion, and at best indirect metabolic information. In close to 100% of MCA territory strokes, SPECT reveals a focally reduced tracer uptake, the extent of which is proportional to the severity of neurological deficit. Defects in tracer uptake almost invariably predict persistent MCA occlusion with subsequent large or malignant infarction when severe and extensive (Giubilei et al., 1990; Berrouschot et al., 1998a; Mahagne et al., 2000), but carry a variable outcome and are exceptionally associated with subsequent death when mild or moderate (Giubilei et al., 1990; Davis et al., 1993; Hanson et al., 1993; Limburg et al., 1990; Marchal et al., 2000).

Using ^{99m}Tc-HMPAO SPECT, Shimosegawa (1994), reported an infarction threshold uptake of 60% of contralateral value, while Nakano et al. (2000) found a threshold about 50% with ^{99m}Tc-ECD. Using a quantitative technique, Umemura et al. (2000) found that tissue with CBF less than 20 mls/100 g.min always evolved to infarction even despite thrombolysis. Massively reduced ^{99m}Tc-HMPAO uptake predicts massive hemorrhagic transformation (Ueda et al., 1994) or no reflow (Herderschee et al., 1991) following therapeutic thrombolysis. Normal or mildly increased uptake is less frequently observed than decreased uptake, but is invariably associated with reversible neurological deficits (Giubilei et al., 1990; Hanson et al., 1993; Berrouschot et al., 1998a; Marchal et al., 2000). Occasional areas of very high tracer uptake ("hot-spots") seem predictive of subsequent infarction (Shimosegawa et al., 1994) and may represent abnormal blood-brain barrier penetration into severely damaged parenchyma rather than true hyperperfusion (Sperling and Lassen, 1993). Findings with ^{99m}Tc-ECD are almost identical to those with ^{99m}Tc-HMPAO but this tracer appears to carry information about cell homeostasis, which may have some interest when studying acute stroke (Mahagne et al., 2000). Recent studies suggest that imaging of early and late ^{99m}Tc-ECD uptake in acute stroke may provide scans reflecting both perfuson and cell function, respectively (Ogasawara et al., 2001).

Either spontaneous or thrombolysis-induced early reperfusion of previously hypoperfused tissue is associated with good outcome (Barber et al., 1998; Herderschee et al., 1991), and spectacular recovery is associated with complete, extensive reperfusion (Baird et al., 1995). However, when the repeat SPECT is done >36–48 hours after onset, reperfusion may not always indicate good outcome because it may have occurred too late, into already necrotic tissue (Jorgensen et al., 1994).

Studies with Xe-CT in acute MCA territory stroke are entirely consistent with the above findings from PET and SPECT. Thus, patients with normal or near-normal CBF had spontaneous resolution of their deficits, while those with considerably reduced CBF in affected territories developed severe brain edema and herniation (Firlik et al., 1998a,b).

Findings with diffusion-weighted imaging (DWI) and perfusion-weighted imaging (PWI)

Diagnostic value

Because DWI/PWI MR has high spatial resolution and is widely available, it has attracted considerable interest in acute stroke imaging. DWI hyperintensity develops minutes only after onset of ischemia and has proved almost 100% sensitive to detect very early ischemic stroke regardless of size and location, making DWI the most sensitive technique so far (Fisher and Albers, 1999). This is of considerable clinical help as, contrary to CT, DWI allows a positive and very early diagnosis of ischemic stroke (as early as 20 minutes of onset), although it has to be borne in mind that other acute brain conditions such as seizure and encephalitis can occasionally lead to DWI hyperintensity. DWI also permits the detection of multiple strokes (including small and "silent" ones), pointing to the existence of a proximal source of emboli, and to discriminate acute lesions adjacent to chronic infarcts. Also important for management is the diagnosis of mechanism afforded by DWI when combined with PWI and MRA of both neck and intracranial vessels, such as carotid and/or MCA occlusion, cervical artery dissection, distal branch occlusion, perforator stroke, small vessel disease, etc.

DWI lesion

The volume of DWI abnormality correlates well with both admission and outcome neurological deficit as well as with final infarct volume (Baird et al., 2000), which would suggest that the DWI lesion equates with irreversibly damaged tissue. However, it is now well established that, consistent with animal studies (Minematsu et al., 1992), the initial DWI lesion contains not only infarcted but penumbral tissue as well. Kidwell et al. (2000) clearly documented reversal of DWI hyperintensity following thrombolysis of an angiographically documented anterior circulation occlusion. According to several studies, however, there may be a threshold of ADC, below which tissue is irreversibly infarcted (Schlaug et al., 1999; Oppenheim et al., 2001; Rohl et al., 2001), but formal validation is still lacking.

PWI changes and the DWI-PWI "mismatch" (Fig. 2)

PWI maps hemodynamic disturbances, which together with DWI provides important pathophysiological information. A mismatch between hypoperfusion extending over the entire MCA territory but DWI lesion restricted to e.g., the striatocapsular/insular area, is found in up to 70% of patients with acute MCA territory stroke (Baird et al., 1998; Albers et al., 1999) (Fig. 2). Under these conditions, the ischaemic penumbra has been operationally defined as tissue with normal diffusion but reduced perfusion, around the core of diffusion abnormality. This mismatch is suggestive of extensive penumbra, in reference to earlier PET data (see above). However, the "hypoperfused area" as seen by PWI, remains ill defined as some define it with MTT or even time-to-peak maps, others with CBV maps, and still others with CBF maps, whereas in fact only the latter truly reflects perfusion. Indeed, based on basic physiology, it is expected that MTT be abnormally prolonged in brain regions where perfusion pressure is decreased due to proximal occlusion/stenosis but CBF is maintained — i.e., normally autoregulated (Szabo et al., 2001). Likewise, the CBV is expected to increase in still autoregulated vascular bed. Thus, both MTT and CBV abnormalities will overestimate the extent of true hypoperfusion. Regarding CBF, although this is the parameter of choice when studying perfusion, it has to be recalled that hypoperfusion does not equate with penumbra, as the oligemic area is also — albeit less severely — hypoperfused. Thus, the area imaged on PWI is probably a mixture of critical flow reduced below the viability threshold, flow within the penumbra range, and oligaemic flow. Another issue with CBF mapping from T2* bolus tracking concerns the reliability of the measurement, as the quantitative method of Ostergaard et al. (1996) is both difficult to implement and liable to measurement errors, while the semi-quantitative approach based on dividing the MTT image by the CBV image is prone to considerable errors at the voxel level. Accordingly, Parsons et al. (2001) and Rohl et al. (2001) have shown that CBF maps are better suited to identify the penumbra than MTT or CBV. Overall, therefore, it has become clear that it is not possible to directly visualize the penumbra with DWI-PWI since as stated above the DWI abnormality does not equate with the core, nor the PWI with the penumbra. So far, therefore, only retrospective identification of the penumbra has been possible, based on the growth of the DWI abnormality and the contours of the final infarct. Schlaug et al. (1999) found a % CBF value (percentage of contralateral side) of $37 \pm 7\%$ and $12 \pm 3\%$ for the penumbra and the core, respectively, which would yield upper 95% limits of a 50% and 18% respectively. Assuming a normal mean of 50 mls/100 g.min, these relative values would correspond to absolute CBF of ~25 and 9 mls/100 g.min, respectively, which compares well with PET data (see above). These values should now be used prospectively to test their reliability in terms of defining the core and penumbra.

Evolution of changes

Despite these caveats, and consistent with the concept of penumbra, perfusion changes precede the development of lesions in DWI, and spontaneously the area of restricted diffusion often progresses within the region of perfusion abnormality, while some areas of decreased perfusion can remain free of DWI signal change, suggesting oligemia (Baird and Warach, 1998). Expansion of the DWI abnormality into the hypoperfused area takes place only if the proximal arterial occlusion remains, whereas spontaneous or therapeutic re-canalization tends to arrest this process (Barber et al., 1998). Also consistent with the concept of penumbra and the PET findings of Furlan et al. (1996), Beaulieu et al. (1999) showed that despite the increase in DWI lesion volume during the initial week, the neurological deficit improved in all patients who displayed reduction of volume of perfusion deficit; in other words, the hypoperfused area represents functionally impaired but still viable tissue. In approximately 50% of patients, the acute DWI lesion was smaller than the final infarct volume measured on T-2 weighted images after 7 days or later. Consistent with PET data, in some patients, lesions enlarged beyond 24 hours, suggesting that penumbra extended beyond the hyperacute phase in these patients (Baird et al., 1997). Studies that looked for threshold values that would predict progression of hypoperfused tissue into DWI abnormality, as compared to non-progression, reported divergent findings, with ADC being the best predictor in some studies (Oppenheim et al., 2001), but CBF in others (Parsons et al., 2001; Rohl et al., 2001), while models combining both DWI and PWI information or CBF and CBV thresholds have been advocated by Wu et al. (2001), and Grandin et al. (2001), respectively.

DWI-PWI Patterns

As found with PET, some patients do not exhibit "mismatch", but rather either a more or less extensive area of matched DWI abnormality and PWI hypoperfusion, suggesting completed infarction, or a DWI abnormality without change in PWI, suggesting early spontaneous recanalization (Warach et al., 1995; Sorensen et al., 1997; Barber et al., 1998; Albers et al., 1999; Oppenheim et al., 2000). A very small fraction of patients exhibit no significant abnormality either with DWI or with PWI, possibly reflecting transient ischemia with short lasting subsequent hyperperfusion, or a non-ischemic process (e.g., migraine).

Implications for therapy

Implications for general management

Demonstration of high OEF or "mismatch" in the setting of acute stroke implies that the autoregulation of CBF is superseded in the affected territory.

Thus, any lowering of the systemic arterial pressure (SAP) is likely to further reduce the CPP and in turn the CBF in the affected tissue, which can be harmful not only for the penumbra — which may precipitate into necrosis-, but also for the oligemia — which may become penumbral and thus in turn at-risk. Accordingly, reductions in SAP in acute stroke have frequently been associated with worse outcome (Ahmed et al., 2000). This issue is especially important in view of the frequent occurrence of reactive hypertension in this setting. Conversely, observing hyperperfusion with low OEF, and particularly if early edema is demonstrated by CT or MRI, may provide rationale for treating excessive arterial hypertension as some experimental studies suggest that hyperperfusion in necrotic tissue may promote the development of malignant brain swelling.

Implications for specific therapy and trials

Based on the data reviewed above, physiologic imaging would help to depict each patient's pathophysiological situation before aggressive therapy is considered. The following framework might be considered: *i*) if early spontaneous recanalization is documented, outcome is invariably good so that no aggressive therapy should be considered; *ii*) if early extensive necrosis is documented, outcome is invariably poor, with considerable risk of massive brain swelling and early death, so that any treatment is likely to fail apart perhaps those directed against vasogenic edema such as surgical brain decompression; and *iii*) if substantial penumbra (i.e. "mismatch") is documented, management should aim at saving as much penumbra as possible, and thus this pattern includes the best candidates for thrombolysis, neuroprotection or both combined. However, demonstration of an area of profoundly decreased function — almost invariably seen after about 6 hrs — places the patient at high risk of hemorrhagic transformation with thrombolysis, so neuroprotection alone should be contemplated, provided it has no SAP reduction side-effect. Specifically designed trials should now test whether incorporating physiologic imaging into the management flow-chart of acute stroke has significant benefit despite the additional time required to perform the procedure. Likewise, pathophysiological heterogeneity suggests that pathophysiologically blind inclusion of acute stroke patients into trials may blur any beneficial effects of the agent being tested. However, whether adding physiologic imaging would result in improved sensitivity of therapeutic trials needs to be tested in its own right.

Finally, the observation that although some patients very early exhibit extensive tissue necrosis or conversely complete reperfusion, penumbra is seen up to 16 hrs in others, suggesting that the therapeutic window needs to be considered in each case (Baron et al., 1995). The positive results of the PRO-ACT II trial of intra-arterial thrombolysis performed up to 6 hrs after onset in a selected sample of patients with documented MCA stem occlusion (Furlan et al., 1999) further strengthens the notion that in a subset of patients there is some tissue still at-risk of infarction hours into the pathologic process.

References

Ackerman RH, Correia JA, Alpert NM, Baron JC, Gouliamos A, Grotta JC, Brownell GL, Taveras JM (1981) Positron imaging in ischemic stroke disease using compounds labeled with oxygen-15. Arch Neurol 38: 537–543

Ahmed N, Nasman P, Wahlgren NG (2000) Effects of intravenous nimodipine on blood pressure and outcome after stroke. Stroke 31: 1250–1255

Albers GW (1999) Expanding the window for thrombolytic therapy in acute stroke. The potential role of acute MRI for patient selection. Stroke 30: 2230–2237

Astrup J, Siesjö BK, Symon L (1981) Thresholds in cerebral ischemia: the ischemic penumbra. Stroke 12: 723–725

Baird AE, Warach S (1998) Magnetic resonance imaging in acute stroke. J Cereb Blood Flow Metabol 18: 583–609

Baird AE, Donnan GA, Austin MC, MacKay WJ (1995) Early reperfusion in the "spectacular shrinking deficit" demonstrated by single-photon emission computed tomography. Neurology 45: 1335–1339

Baird AE, Benfield A, Schlaug G, Siewert B, Lovblad KO, Edelman RR, Warach S (1997) Enlargement of human cerebral ischemic lesion volumes measured by diffusion-weighted magnetic resonance imaging. Ann Neurol 41: 581–589

Baird AE, Lövblad KO, Dashe JF, Connor A, Burzynski C, Schlaug G, Straroselskaya, Edelman R, Warach S (2000) Clinical correlations of diffusion and perfusion lesion volumes in acute ischemic stroke. Cerebrovasc Dis 10: 441–448

Barber PA, Davis SM, Darby DG, Desmond PM, Gerraty RP, Yang Q, Donnan GA, Tress BM (1999) Absent middle cerebral artery flow predicts the presence and evolution of the ischemic penumbra. Neurology 52: 1125–1132

Baron JC (1999) Mapping the ischaemic penumbra with PET: implications for acute stroke treatment. Cerebrovasc Dis 9: 193–201

Baron JC (2001) Mapping the ischaemic penumbra with PET: a new approach. Brain 124: 2–4

Baron JC, Marchal G (2000) Functional imaging in vascular disorders. In: Mazziotta et al (eds) Brain mapping: the disorders. Academic Press, San Diego, pp 299–316

Baron JC, Bousser MG, Comar D, et al (1981) Non invasive tomographic study of cerebral blood flow and oxygen metabolism in vivo: potentials, limitations and clinical applications in cerebral ischemic disorders. Eur Neurol 20: 273–284

Baron JC, Bousser MG, Rey A, et al (1981) Reversal of focal "misery-perfusion syndrome" by extra-intracranial arterial bypass in hemodynamic cerebral ischemia: a case study with $^{15}0$ positron tomography. Stroke 12: 454–459

Baron JC, Frackowiak RSJ, Herholz K, et al (1989) Use of positron emission tomography in the investigation of cerebral hemodynamics and energy metabolism in cerebrovascular disease. J Cereb Blood Flow Metab 9: 723–742

Baron JC, von Kummer R, Del Zoppo, GJ (1995) Treatment of acute ischemic stroke: challenging the concept of a rigid and universal time window. Stroke 26: 2219–2221

Beaulieu C, et al (1999) Longitudinal magnetic resonance imaging study of perfusion and diffusion in stroke: evolution of lesion volume and correlation with clinical outcome. Ann Neurol 46: 568–578

Berrouschot J, Barthel H, von Kummer R, et al (1998) 99 m technetium-ethyl-cysteinate-dimer single-photon emission CT can predict fatal ischemic brain edema. Stroke 12: 2556–2562

Berrouschot J, Barthel H, Hesse S, et al (1998) Differentiation between transient ischemic attack and ischemic stroke within the first six hours after onset of symtoms by using 99mTc-ECD-SPECT. J Cereb Blood Flow Metab 18: 921–929

Calamante F, et al (1999) Measuring cerebral blood flow using magnetic resonance imaging techniques. J Cereb Blood Flow Metab 19: 701–735

Firlik AD, Rubin G, Yonas H, Wechsler LR (1998a) Relation between cerebral blood flow and neurologic deficit resolution in acute ischemic stroke. Neurology 51: 177–182
Firlik AD, Yonas H, Kaufmann AM, Wechsler LR, Jungreis CA, Fukui MB, Williams RL (1998b) Relationship between cerebral blood flow and the development of swelling and life-threatening herniation in acute ischemic stroke. J Neurosurg 89: 243–249
Fisher M, Albers GW (1999) Application of diffusion-perfusion MRI in acute ischemic stroke. Neurology 52: 1750–1756
Furlan M, Marchal G, Viader F, et al (1996) Spontaneous neurological recovery after stroke and the fate of the ischemic penumbra. Ann Neurol 40: 216–226
Furlan A, Higashida R, Wechsler L, Gent M, Rowley H, Kase C, Pessin M, Ahuja A, Callahan F, Clark WM, Silver F, Rivera F (1999) Intra-arterial prourokinase for acute ischemic stroke. The PROACT II study: a randomized controlled trial. JAMA 282: 2003–2011
Gillard JH, Barker PB, Van Zijl PC, Bryan RN, Oppenheimer SM (1996) Proton MR spectroscopy in acute middle cerebral artery stroke. Am J Neuroradiol 17: 873–886
Ginsberg MD, Bogousslavsky J (eds) (1998) Cerebrovascular diseases. Blackwell Science, New York, 2067 pp
Giubilei F, Lenzi GL, Di Piero V, et al (1990) Predictive value of brain perfusion single-photon emission computed tomography in acute ischemic stroke. Stroke 21: 895–900
Grandin, Duprez TP, Smith AM, Mataigne F, Peeters A, Oppenheim C, Cosnard G (2001) Usefulness of magnetic resonance-derived quantitative measurements of cerebral blood flow and volume in prediction of infarct growth in hyperacute stroke. Stroke 32: 1147–1153
Heiss WD, Huber M, Fink GR, Herholz K, Pietryk U, Wagner R, Wienhard K (1992) Progressive derangement of periinfarct viable tissue in ischemic stroke. J Cereb Blood Flow Metab 12: 193–203
Heiss WD, Graf R, Löttgen J, Ohta K, Fujita T, Wagner R, Grond M, Wienhard K (1997) Repeat positron emission tomographic studies in transient middle cerebral artery occlusion in cats: residual perfusion and efficacy of postischemic reperfusion. J Cereb Blood Flow Metab 17: 388–400
Heiss WD, Grond M, Thiel A, Von Stockhausen HM, Rudolf J, Ghaemi M, Löttgen J, Stenzel C, Pawlik G (1998a) Tissue at risk of infarction rescued by early reperfusion: a positron emission tomography study in systemic recombinant tissue plasminogen activator thrombolysis of acute stroke. J Cereb Blood Flow Metab 18: 1298–1307
Heiss WD, Grond M, Thiel A, Ghaemi M, Sobesky J, Rudolf J, Bauer B, Wienhard K (1998b) Permanent cortical damage detected by flumazenil positron emission tomography in acute stroke. Stroke 29: 454–461
Heiss W-D, Thiel A, Grond M, et al (1999) Which targets are relevant for therapy of acute ischemic stroke? Stroke 30: 1486–1489
Heiss WD, Kracht L, Grond M, Rudolf J, Bauer B, Wienhard K, et al (2000) Early 11C-flumazenil/H2O positron emission tomography predicts irreversible ischemic cortical damage in stroke patients receiving acute thrombolytic therapy. Stroke 31: 366–369
Heiss WD, Kracht LW, Thiel A, Grond M, Pawlik G (2001) Penumbral probability thresholds of cortical flumazenil binding and blood flow predicting tissue outcome in patients with cerebral ischaemia. Brain 124: 20–29
Heiss W-D, Forsting M, Diener H-C (2001) Imaging in cerebrovascular diseases. Curr Opin Neurol 14: 67–75
Jones TH, Morawetz RE, Crowell RM, et al (1981) Thresholds of focal cerebral ischaemia in awake monkeys. J Neurosurg 54: 773–782
Kamada K, Saguer M, Möller M, Wicklow K, Katenhäuser M, Kober H, Vieth J (1997) Functional and metabolic analysis of cerebral ischemia using magnetoencephalography and proton magnetic resonance spectroscopy. Ann Neurol 42: 554–563
Kidwell C, Saver J, Mattiello J, et al (2000) Thrombolytic reversal of acute human cerebral ischaemic injury shown by diffusion/perfusion magnetic resonance imaging. Ann Neurol 47: 462–469

Lassen NA (1966) The luxury perfusion syndrome and its possible relation to acute metabolic acidosis localised within the brain. Lancet ii: 1113–1115
Mahagne MH, Darcourt J, Migneco O, Fournier JP, Ducoeur S, Thiercelin D, Bertrand F, Bussière F, Chatel M, Baron JC (2000) Early 99mTc-ECD brain SPECT in the acute phase of stroke: a strong predictor of neurological recovery. Cerebrovasc Dis 10: 364–373
Marchal G, Serrati C, Rioux P, et al (1993) PET imaging of cerebral perfusion and oxygen consumption in acute ischaemic stroke: relation to outcome. Lancet 341: 925–927
Marchal G, Rioux P, Serrati C, et al (1995) Value of acute-stage PET in predicting neurological outcome after ischemic stroke: further assessment. Stroke 26: 524–525
Marchal G, Beaudouin V, Rioux P, et al (1996) Prolonged persistence of substantial volumes of potentially viable brain tissue after stroke: a correlative PET-CT study with voxel-based data analysis. Stroke 27: 599–606
Marchal G, Furlan M, Beaudouin V, et al (1996) Early spontaneous hyperperfusion after stroke: a marker of favorable tissue outcome? Brain 119: 409–419
Marchal G, Benali K, Iglesias S, et al (1999a) Voxel-based mapping of irreversible tissue damage by PET in the acute stage of ischemic stroke. Brain 123: 2387–2400
Marchal G, Young AR, Baron JC (1999b) Early post-ischaemic hyperperfusion: pathophysiological insights from positron emission tomography. J Cereb Blood Flow Metab 19: 467–482
Marchal G, Bouvard G, Iglesias S, Sebastien B, Benali K, Defer G, Viader F, Baron JC (2000) Predictive value of 99mTc-HMPAO for neurological outcome/recovery in the acute stage of stroke. Cerebrovasc Dis 10: 8–17
Minematsu K, et al (1992) Reversible focal ischemic injury demonstrated by diffusion-weighted magnetic resonance imaging in rats. Stroke 23: 1304–1310
Nakano S, Iseda T, Ikeda T, Yoneyama T, Wakisaka S (2000) Thresholds of ischemia salvageable with intravenous tissue plasminogen activator therapy: evaluation with cerebral blood flow single-photon emission computed tomographic measurements. Neurosurgery 47: 68–73
Ogasawara K, Ogawa A, Konno H, Shibanai K, Doi M, Kuroda K, Yoshimoto T (2001) Combination of early and delayed SPET imaging using technetium-99m ethyl cysteinate dimer immediately after local intra-arterial thrombolysis. Eur J Nucl Med 28: 498–505
Oppenheim C, Samson Y, Manai R, Lalam T, Vandamme X, Crozier S, Srour A, Cornu P, Dormont D, Rancurel G, Marsault C (2000) Prediction of malignant middle cerebral artery infarction by diffusion-weighted imaging. Stroke 31: 2175–2181
Oppenheim C, Grandin C, Samson Y, Smith A, Duprez T, Marsault C, Cosnard G (2001) Is there an apparent diffusion coefficient threshold in predicting tissue viability in hyperacute stroke? Stroke 32: 2486–2491
Ostergaard L, Weisskoff RM, Chesler DA, Gyldensted C, Rosen BR (1996) High resolution measurement of cerebral blood flow using intravascular tracer bolus passages. I. Mathematical approach and statistical analysis. Magn Res Med 36: 715–725
Parsons MW, Yang Q, Barber A, Darby DG, Desmond PM, Gerraty RP, Tress BM, Davis SM (2001) Perfusion magnetic resonance imaging maps in hyperacute stroke. Relative cerebral blood flow most accurately identifies tissue destined to infarct. Stroke 32: 1581–1587
Ramsay SC, Weiller C, Myers R, et al (1992) Monitoring by PET of macrophage accumulation in brain after ischaemic stroke. Lancet 239: 1054–1055
Read SJ, Hirano T, Abbott DF, et al (1998) Identifying hypoxic tissue after acute ischemic stroke using PET and 18F-fluoromisonidazole. Neurology 51: 1617–1621
Read SJ, Hirano T, Abbott DF, Markus R, Sachinidis JI, Tochon-Danguy HJ, Chan JG, Egan GF, Scott AM, Bladin CF, McKay WJ, Donnan GA (2000) The fate of hypoxic

tissue on ^{18}F-fluoromisonidazole positron emission tomography after ischemic stroke. Ann Neurol 48: 228–235

Røhl L, Østergaard, Simonsen CZ, Vestergaard-Poulsen P, Andersen G, Sakoh M, Le Bihan D, Gyldensted C (2001) Viability thresholds of ischemic penumbra of hyperacute stroke defined by perfusion-weighted MRI and apparent diffusion coefficient. Stroke 32: 1140–1146

Schlaug G, et al (1997) Time course of the apparent diffusion coefficient (ADC) abnormality in human stroke. Neurology 49: 113–119

Schlaug G, et al (1999) The ischemic penumbra: operationally defined by diffusion and perfusion MRI. Neurology 53: 1528–1537

Senda M, Alpert NM, Mackay BC, Buxton RB, Correia JA, Weise SB, Ackerman RH, Dorer D, Buonanno FS (1989) Evaluation of the $^{11}CO2$ positron emission tomographic method for measuring brain pH.II. Quantitative pH mapping in patients with ischemic cerebrovascular diseases. J Cereb Blood Flow Metabol 9: 859–873

Sette G, Baron JC, Young AR, et al (1993) In vivo mapping of brain benzodiazepine receptor changes by positron emission tomography after focal ischemia in the anesthetized baboon. Stroke 24: 2046–2058

Shimosegawa E, Hatazawa J, Inugami A, et al (1994) Cerebral infarction within six hours of onset: prediction of completed infarction with technetium-99m-HMPAO SPECT. J Nucl Med 35: 1097–1103

Sorensen AG, Buonanno FS, Gonzalez RG, Schwamm LH, Lev MH, Huang-Hellinger FR, Reese TG, Weisskoff RM, Da'vis TL, Suwanwela N, Can U, Moreira JA, Copen WA, Look RB, Finklestein SP, Rosen BR, Koroshetz WJ (1996) Hyperacute stroke: evaluation with combined multisection diffusion-weighted and hemodynamically weighted echo-planar MR imaging. Radiology 199: 391–401

Sperling B, Lassen NA (1993) Hyperfixation of HMPAO in subacute ischemic stroke leading to spuriously high estimates of cerebral blood flow by SPECT. Stroke 24: 193–194

Syrota A, Samson Y, Boullais C, Wajnberg P, Loc'h C, Crouzel C, Maziere B, Soussaline F, Baron JC (1985) Tomographic mapping of brain intracellular pH and extracellular water space in stroke patients. J Cereb Blood Flow Metabol 5: 358–385

Szabo K, Kern R, Gass A, Hirsch J, Hennerici M (2001) Acute stroke patterns in patients with internal carotid artery disease. A diffusion-weighted magnetic resonance imaging study. Stroke 32: 1323–1329

Thijs VN, Adami A, Neumann-Haefelin T, Moseley ME, Marks MP, Albers GW (2001) Relationship between severity of MR perfusion deficit and DWI lesion evolution. Neurology 57: 1205–1211

Touzani O, Young AR, Derlon J-M, Beaudouin V, Marchal G, Rioux P, Mézenge F, Baron JC, MacKenzie ET (1995) Sequential studies of severely hypometabolic tissue volumes after permanent middle cerebral artery occlusion. A positron emission tomographic investigation in anesthetized baboons. Stroke 26: 2112–2119

Touzani O, Young AR, Derlon JM, et al (1997) Progressive impairment of brain oxidative metabolism reversed by reperfusion following middle cerebral artery occlusion in anaesthetized baboons. Brain Res 767: 17–25

Ueda T, Hatakeyama T, Kumon Y, et al (1994) Evaluation of risk of hemorrhagic transformation in local intra-arterial thrombolysis in acute ischemic stroke by initial SPECT. Stroke 25: 298–303

Warach S, et al (1992) Fast magnetic resonance diffusion-weighted imaging of acute human stroke. Neurology 42: 1717–1723

Warach S, et al (1995) Acute human stroke studied by whole brain echo planar diffusion-weighted magnetic resonance imaging. Ann Neurol 37: 231–241

Wise RJS, Bernardi S, Frackowiak RSJ, et al (1983) Serial observations on the pathophysiology of acute stroke. The transition from ischaemia to infarction as reflected in regional oxygen extraction. Brain 106: 197–222

Wu O, Koroshetz WJ, Østergaard L, Buonanno FS, Copen WA, Gonzalez G, Rordorf G, Rosen BR, Schwamm LH, Weisskoff RM, Sorensen AG (2001) Predicting tissue outcome in acute human cerebral ischemia using combined diffusion — and perfusion-weighted MR imaging. Stroke 32: 933–942

Young AR, Touzani O, Derlon JM, Sette G, MacKenzie ET, Baron JC (1997) Early reperfusion in the anesthetized baboon reduces brain damage following middle cerebral artery occlusion. Stroke 28: 632–638

Author's address: Prof. J.-C. Baron, Department of Neurology, Addenbrooke's Hospital, Box 83, Cambridge CB2 2QQ, United Kingdom, e-mail: jcb54@cam.ac.uk

J Neural Transm (2002) [Suppl] 63: 37–57

Stroke — acute interventions

W.-D. Heiss

Max-Planck-Institut für neurologische Forschung and Neurologische Universitätsklinik, Köln, Federal Republic of Germany

Summary. The reduction of blood flow to parts of the brain is the cause of ischemic stroke leading to functional deficits and, if prolonged, to irreversible neurological and morphological defects. The fast reperfusion, therefore is the most important therapeutic strategy and was proven to be effective in clinical trials. Steps to intervene with secondary biochemical, molecular, or inflammatory disturbances were not successful so far. Since direct therapeutic interventions are limited, the general management of the stroke victim is of utmost importance — and was shown to be most successful in dedicated stroke units.

Acute therapeutic interventions in ischemic stroke can only be successful as long as tissue in the area of the ischemic compromise is still viable. The area of irreversible damage can be identified and distinguished from the penumbral zone, i.e., tissue with impaired function but preserved morphology by functional imaging modalities, like positron emission tomography (PET) or perfusion-(PW) and diffusion-weighted (DW) magnetic resonance imaging (MRI). In such studies it was demonstrated that a large portion of the final infarct is irreversibly affected in the first few hours in many patients. A considerable tissue volume is viable but critically hypoperfused; a smaller portion of the final infarct is sufficiently perfused and in this area secondary and delayed biochemical and molecular mechanisms contribute to the damage. Based on this concept the improvement of perfusion within the time window of opportunity must be the primary goal in treatment of ischemic stroke, and neuroprotective and other strategies can only play a supportive and additive role. That this is the case can be seen from the results of many controlled therapeutic trials, in which up to now only thrombolytic therapy with a 3h time window for systemic and a 6h time window for intraarterial application proved its efficacy, whereas all trials with neuroprotective, anti-inflammatory or anti-apoptotic strategies failed. Since the direct treatment strategies are limited the acute management of stroke victims is of utmost importance: This can be achieved optimally in dedicated stroke units in which the outcome was significantly improved over the regular care. It is still to be investigated if invasive strategies — e.g., craniectomy and hypothermia — or the combination of reperfusion and neuroprotective therapy can improve the outcome after ischemic stroke.

Introduction

The acute management of ischemic stroke must be based on the pathophysiological mechanisms leading to tissue damage. Despite considerable progress has been made in recent years in the understanding of the time course of pathophysiological events contributing and finally leading to infarction (Barone and Feuerstein, 1999) the search for effective interventions to prevent this damage has been discouraging (Grotta, 1994). The cascade of biochemical and molecular changes involved in ischemic damage is initiated by the disturbance of flow, and therefore the primary strategy must be the restoration of a sufficient perfusion. This predominant therapeutic goal could be supported by measures interfering with the biochemical and molecular changes contributing to neuronal damage. A necessary prerequisite for any intervention is the existence of functionally impaired but viable and potentially salvageable tissue, since irreversibly damaged tissue cannot benefit from any strategy, and forced reperfusion could even be detrimental by causing hemorrhage and enhancing edema. The perfusional condition of tissue is therefore of utmost importance in the early time after a stroke.

Rationale for effective treatment in stroke

Severity and extent of the ischemic compromise can be clearly assessed in experimental models for which flow thresholds for preservation of function and morphology were defined (review in (Heiss and Graf, 1994; Hossmann, 1994). Ischemic tissue is only amenable to therapy as long as the lack of blood supply did not lead to morphological destruction and only caused functional impairment. This tissue, termed the *penumbra* (Astrup et al., 1981), is perfused at a level within the thresholds of functional impairment and morphological integrity and has the capacity to recover if perfusion is improved. The extent of this tissue compartment is dependent on residual flow and duration of flow disturbance: It can be clearly demonstrated in animal experiments with permanent and transient occlusion of cerebral vessels (Heiss et al., 2001a) that the volume of functionally impaired but morphologically intact tissue is large and involves even the center of the vascular territory with impaired blood supply immediately after the onset of the perfusional disturbance, and it becomes progressively smaller with time elapsed since the vascular attack. This concept as developed in animal experiments defines the penumbra as a dynamic process depending on residual perfusion and duration, with conversion into irreversible neuronal damage over time, progressing from the center of dense ischemia to the surrounding tissue with less severe but still critical hypoperfusion. This concept explains the *time window of therapeutic opportunity*: it is very short for the core of ischemia and may extend to several hours in the moderately hypoperfused adjacent areas.

In the clinical setting of acute stroke management the assessment of the condition of the ischemically affected tissue is extremely difficult and necessitates logistically complex and expensive investigative procedures, which cannot be performed routinely. Studies performed in selected cases with determination of regional cerebral blood flow (rCBF), regional cerebral consumption of oxygen ($rCMO_2$), regional oxygen extraction fraction (rOEF), and regional cerebral metabolic rate for glucose ($rCMR_{glc}$) by positron emission tomography (PET) have broadened the knowledge of pathophysiological mechanisms leading to ischemic infarction and in some instances could explain the success or failure of therapeutic interventions. In individual cases, disturbances of flow and energy metabolism in the acute stage could be related to the final fate of the tissue: synchronous decreases of flow and oxygen consumption below threshold values predicted infarction, whereas uncoupled decreases of flow with oxygen consumption preserved at a higher value (termed "misery perfusion" by (Baron et al., 1981) indicated tissue with uncertain prognosis, i.e. the potential for recovery or necrosis. The determination of absolute values of thresholds in patients, however, is difficult since the necessary calculation require arterial blood sampling. Additionally, measurements of tracer concentrations are affected by considerable variability causing especially high statistical errors at low count rates. As a consequence, the reported values for the threshold of morphological damage and of the upper limit of penumbra given by different authors vary considerably (review in Heiss, 2000). These values are also affected by the time of determination after the vascular attack since the variability of flow in the course after the attack which has a considerable effect on outcome cannot be assessed. For preservation of morphology the necessary oxygen consumption was determined to be around 65 μmol/100 g/min, the flow thresholds ranged between 5 and 12 ml/100 g/min. For the upper limit of the penumbra flow values between 14 and 22 ml/100 g/min were reported. These values corresponded to those assessed by other methods as perfusion weighted magnetic resonance imaging (PW-MRI), single photon emission computed tomography (SPECT), and Xe-enhanced computed tomography (Xe-CT).

Using flow values measured in the first hours after a stroke *various compartments* of tissue and their contribution to the final infarct on CT/MRI can be determined. When the threshold for probable infarction was arbitrarily set to the conventional value of 12 ml/100 g/min and that for the upper limit of penumbra to 18 ml/100 g/min (Hakim et al., 1987) a large compartment of the final infarct (70%) was critically perfused, i.e. at a level predicting necrosis; a smaller compartment (18%) had flow values in the penumbra range and a fairly small compartment (12%) was sufficiently perfused (Heiss et al., 1999). This result carries important implications for treatment of acute stroke: a significant effect can only be achieved if perfusion is improved before irreversible damage has occurred.

The determination of rCBF is an unreliable predictor for the assessment of *irreversible damage*. For that purpose quantitative measurement of $CMRO_2$ and CBF is necessary requiring arterial blood sampling which is prohibited when invasive strategies, e.g. thrombolysis, are planned. Therefore, a marker of neuronal integrity is needed which can noninvasively distinguish between viable and irreversibly damaged neurons. As such tracers labeled ligands of central benzodiazepine receptors can be applied which reliably differentiated infarcted from non-infarcted cortex in animal experiments and in stroke patients (Heiss et al., 2001b). Using 11C-flumazenil as a marker of neuronal integrity and $H_2{}^{15}O$ for flow determinations, the pathophysiological changes early after ischemic stroke could be more accurately specified: 55% of the volume of the final infarct had FMZ uptake decreased below the limit of 95% probability for infarction at the study in the first hours after stroke; 21% of the final infarct had flow below 14 ml/100 g/min, the 95% probability threshold for survival, but FMZ above the critical value, thereby indicating penumbra tissue. Only 13% of the final infarct exhibited neuronal integrity and CBF values above the penumbral range. These results stress again the crucial role of early reperfusion in the treatment of ischemic stroke. Only a rather small compartment is initially viable and sufficiently perfused, but eventually becomes necrotic mainly owing to delayed mechanisms; only this tissue volume may benefit from neuroprotective or other measures exclusively targeted to secondary damage.

Controlled multitracer trials with thrombolysis

Cerebral angiography conducted soon after the onset of stroke demonstrates arterial occlusion in up to 80 percent of acute infarctions (Fieschi et al., 1989; del Zoppo et al., 1992). Thrombolytic recanalization of occluded arteries therefore may reduce the degree of injury to the brain if it is done before the process of infarction has been completed. Since intracerebral hemorrhage was a frequent major complication reported in early trials of thrombolytic therapy (Wardlaw et al., 1997) the use of recombinant human tissue plasminogen activator (rt-PA) for cerebral arterial thrombolysis required careful evaluation of both, the risks and the potential benefits in controlled randomized multitracer trials.

ECASS I

In ECASS I, 620 patients were randomized and treated within 6 hours from the onset of symptoms (Hacke et al., 1995). The dose of rt-PA was 1.1 mg/kg body weight up to 100 mg. A bolus of 10% of the total dose was injected intravenously within 1–2 min followed by the rest of the dose as an intravenous infusion lasting 1 hour. The primary predetermined endpoints were Barthel Index (BI) and modified Rankin Scale (mRS) at day 90. Patients who died received the worst score in BI and mRS. The occurrence of large parenchymatous hemorrhages was significantly more frequent in the rt-PA-treated patients (19.8% v. 6.5%). No significant difference was seen between rt-PA and placebo in the primary outcome events due to increased mortality of rt-PA-treated patients at day 90 compared with placebo-treated patients (22.4 vs. 15.8%). If the results of ECASS I had been analyzed based on the NINDS methodology of dichotomized outcomes, ECASS I would have been a positive trial.

NINDS

The NINDS rt-PA Stroke Study Group enrolled and treated 624 patients within 3 hours of the onset of symptoms, half of them within 90 min (The NINDS rt-PA Stroke Study Group, 1995). The dose of rt-PA was 0.9 mg/kg body weight (maximum 90 mg), 10% of which was given as a bolus followed by delivery of the remaining 90% as a constant infusion over a period of 60 min. It assessed the clinical outcome according to BI, mRS, Glasgow Outcome Scale and National Institute of Health Stroke Scale. In the NINDS trial, 11–13% more patients in the rt-PA arm reached an excellent functional outcome with no increase in mortality, although symptomatic hemorrhages were increased tenfold by thrombolysis (6.4 vs. 0.6%). On the basis of the results, rt-PA was approved in the US for use within a 3-hour time window.

ECASS II

In ECASS II, 800 patients were randomized and treated. The dose was the same as in the NINDS trial, 0.9 mg/kg, and ECASS II included a strict blood pressure control and a 6-hour time window (Hacke et al., 1998). The primary endpoint was the proportion of patients with favorable outcome (mRS 0–1). All investigators were trained to read baseline CTs. In ECASS I, 8.6% of patients had infarcts larger than one third of the MCA territory, while in ECASS II, such protocol violations only occurred in 4.6% of patients. Mortality of the ECASS II rt-PA arm was 10.3% and that of the placebo arm 10.7%, despite a 2.5-fold increase in symptomatic parenchymal hemorrhages after rt-PA therapy (8.8 vs. 3.4%). ECASS II was powered to detect a 10% effect size in the primary endpoint based on the data from ECASS I and the NINDS trial. This primary outcome event was not reached, probably due to extremely good outcome in the placebo group (36.6% of the patients in the placebo group and 40.3% in the rt-PA group reached modified Rankin scale 0–1 at 3 months). However, a post hoc analysis applying a more often used dichotomization for independent versus dead or dependent patients revealed a significant 8.3% difference favoring rt-PA therapy (54.3 vs. 46.0%), which is equivalent to 83 per 1,000 fewer patients dead or disabled after thrombolysis.

A recent follow-up study of the NINDS trial demonstrated a sustained benefit of rt-PA at 12 months (Kwiatkowski et al., 1999). Donnan (in Hacke et al., 1999) was the first to present a meta-analysis of the three trials, ECASS I, the NINDS trial and ECASS II. It revealed that thrombolysis decreases the risk of death and dependency. For each 1,000 patients treated within 3 hours, there will be 140 less dead or dependent and 90 less, if the treatment is given within 6 hours. A recent Cochrane systematic review verified Donnan's analysis, and also revealed that it is possible to reduce the number of dead and disabled stroke patients with thrombolysis (Wardlaw et al., 2000). These data support the view that rt-PA should be part of the management of acute ischemic stroke within 3 hours, and probably beyond in selected patients and experienced centers (The European Ad Hoc Consensus Group, 1996). It was demonstrated that intra-arterial application of a thrombolytic agent (prourokinase) is efficient up to 6h after the attack, if angiography reveals occlusion of a major vessel (Furlan et al., 1999). It was also suggested repeatedly (Kaste, 2001), that neuroprotective agents may prolong the time interval that the brain can tolerate ischemia before reperfusion and thereby extend the time window for thrombolysis.

Experience with routine application of rtPA in acute ischemic stroke

Since its approval by the FDA in 1996 rtPA has been used safely and effectively in routine clinical practice in academic medical centers as well as in community hospitals, and guidelines have been developed to ensure safety in the use of rtPA for acute ischemic stroke (Adams et al., 1996). These guidelines restrict the routine use of rtPA to those patients who can be treated within 3h of symptom onset and emphasize the importance of involving physicians with expertise in the diagnosis of stroke, in the interpretation of CT scans and in the ability to handle hemorrhagic complications. Up to now, 7 studies on routine use have been published (Grond et al., 1998; Chiu et al., 1998; Trouillas et al., 1998; Schmülling et al., 2000; Albers et al., 2000; Katzan et al., 2000; Wang et al., 2000; Chapman et al., 2000) and one large survey has been presented (Tanne et al., 2000). In order to increase the number of patients who can benefit from rtPA treatment a referral system must be organized to transfer appropriate cases in the early hours after ischemic stroke to the appropriate centers. Such referral systems were successfully set up for urban (Grond et al., 1998) as well as for rural environments (Davenport et al., 2000). With the exception of one study (Katzan et al., 2000) in which exclusion criteria were not carefully followed, all the published experience supports the beneficial effect of rtPA treatment (Hacke et al., 1999) but also stress the point that only a small portion (1–2%) of all patients with acute ischemic stroke are actually receiving this potentially effective therapy.

The experience in our center, where more than 300 patients with acute ischemic stroke received rtPA intravenously within 3h after symptom onset following the NINDS protocol, is given as an example of thrombolytic treatment in clinical routine. Based on a cooperative referral system involving 14 city hospitals and the emergency system patients with suspected acute ischemic stroke are admitted using age under 80, no severe impairment of consciousness and presentation within 3h of symptom onset as simple selection criteria. Of these preselected cases 22% were receiving iv rtPA treatment within the time window (Grond et al., 1998). The outcomes of patients treated in Cologne were very similar to those of the patients in the NINDS trails, and this effect carries through also for the 150 patients followed up to 12 months after treatment (Schmülling et al., 2000). As demonstrated in the diagrams of Fig. 1, the proportion of patients in the no or minimal disability group (modified Rankin Scale 0 and 1) was comparable (42%) to the NINDS cohort

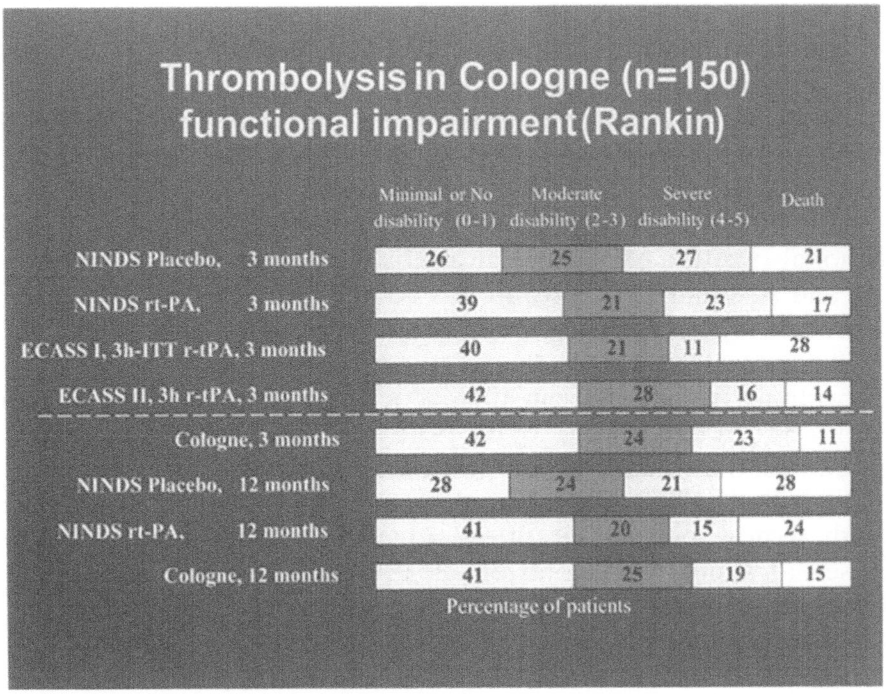

Fig. 1. Modified Rankin Scale scores at 3 and 12 months in patients treated in Cologne compared with patients from NINDS rt-PA Stroke Trial placebo and treatment groups (3 and 12 months) and with the ECASS I and II 3h cohorts (3 months)

as well as the 3h cohort of ECASS I and II after 3 months and to the NINDS cohort (Kwiatkowski et al., 1999) after 12 months (both 41%). The number of deceased patients (11% after 3 months, 15% after 12 months) was the lowest in the Cologne study, but this might be related to the exclusion of very severe cases from this treatment (median NIHSS score at inclusion in Cologne 11 — as in ECASS II —, but 14 for NINDS rtPA trial). Despite the application of heparin after thrombolysis in the majority of patients the rate of symptomatic parenchymal hemorrhages (4%) was similar as in ECASS II, slightly lower than in the NINDS and distinctly lower than in the ECASS I treatment groups. Similar results were reported in surveys collecting data of routinely treated stroke patients from various centers (Chiu et al., 1998; Hacke et al., 1998; Albers, 1999; Tanne et al., 2000; Wang et al., 2000; Chapman et al., 2000).

Effects of thrombolysis on the penumbra

Several small treatment studies used effects on the penumbra, as assessed by functional imaging, as surrogate targets. An effect of the therapeutic intervention can therefore only be expected as long as penumbral tissue is present, and in most instances the compartment of penumbral tissue is rather small at the time of intervention (Heiss et al., 1999). Thrombolysis is still the only approved therapy for acute ischemic stroke, and its effect was demonstrated recently in several imaging studies, in which reperfusion to penumbral tissue was associated with improvement in neurological deficits. Previous SPECT observations on the combined effect of severity of initial hypoperfusion and extent of reperfusion on the final outcome (Sasaki et al., 1996; Ryu et al., 1999; Ueda et al., 1999) were supported by results in a small cohort selected from the National Institute of Neurological Disorders and Stroke (NINDS) study (Grotta and Alexandrov, 1998). In this double-blind controlled study, significantly greater reperfusion occurred in the recombinant tissue-type plasminogen activator-treated patients than in the placebo group.

The volume of tissue salvaged by reperfusion was established in a study in which CBF, as determined by $H_2^{15}O$-PET within 3h of stroke onset, was compared with the volume of infarction determined on MRI 3 weeks after the ictus (Heiss et al., 1998). The percentage of initially critically ischemic voxels (i.e. with a flow below the threshold of 12 ml/100g/min) that became reperfused at almost normal levels clearly predicted the degree of clinical improvement achieved within 3 weeks. Overall, only 22.7% of the grey matter that was initially perfused at rates below the conventional threshold of critical ischemia became necrotic after thrombolytic therapy in this small sample of 12 patients. That means, that a considerable portion of the critically hypoperfused tissue was probably salvaged by the reperfusion therapy. Another PET study in 11 patients (Heiss et al., 2000) indicated that hypoperfused tissue could benefit from reperfusion only as long as cortical flumazenil binding was not reduced to or below 3.4 times the mean uptake in white matter (Fig. 2). This marker of neuronal integrity can therefore serve as an indicator for irreversibly damaged tissue that is not amenable to treatment.

CT perfusion imaging (Klotz and König, 1999; Segal et al., 1999) and Xenon enhanced CT (Rubin et al., 1999) were also used in an attempt to predict outcome after thrombolysis, but a refinement of CT for reliable identification of irreversible tissue damage during the first hours after onset of symptoms is required before these methods can be introduced into clinical routine (Koroshetz and Gonzales, 1999).

Recently, the difference in the volumes of abnormality in PWI and DWI has been used as a surrogate marker of efficacy in stroke trials (Fisher and Albers, 1999; Saver et al., 1999). Two groups reported results of serial DW and PW imaging in patients undergoing intravenous thrombolysis. Inhibition of lesion growth was observed in patients experiencing reperfusion compared with patients with persistent perfusion deficits (Jansen et al., 1999; Schellinger et al., 2000). Normalization of PWI occurred in five out of six patients receiving recombinant tissue-type plasminogen activator, but only in one out of six patients in the control group (Marks et al., 1999). Increases in ADC, which were observed in ischemic zones of five patients with early reperfusion, were closely associated with the reperfusion seen after intravenous recombinant tissue-type plasminogen activator therapy. Similar effects were observed after intra-arterial thrombolytic therapy within 6h of symptom onset (Kidwell et al., 2000). With recanalization proved by angiography, the volume of DWI

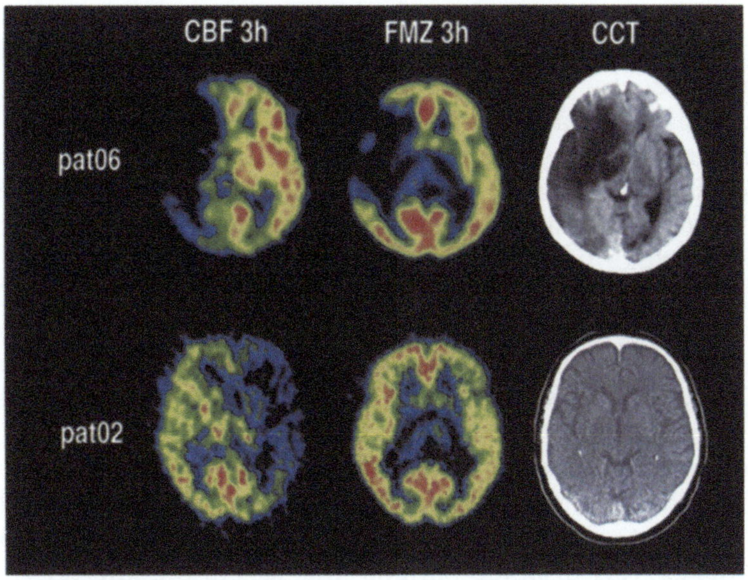

Fig. 2. Effect of rt-PA treatment in two patients with large ischemic areas (white arrows): patient 06 with area of decreased FMZ binding (blue arrow) and corresponding large infarction on late cranial CT (red arrow); patient 02 with no defect in FMZ binding and no infarcted cortex on late cranial CT

lesions decreased from 23 cm^3 at baseline to 10 cm^3 early after lysis. This study demonstrated that perfusion deficits can be resolved and that DWI signatures of early ischemic injury can be reversed by prompt thrombolytic vessel recanalization. This means that the ischemic penumbra includes not only a region of diffusion/perfusion mismatch, but also portions of the volume of initial diffusion abnormality. The various techniques that permit identification of the penumbra (i.e. potentially salvageable tissue) might be applied to extend the window of therapeutic opportunity (Albers, 1999).

Controlled defibrinogenation by ancrod

A therapeutic alternative to the lysis of the thrombotic clot in acute stroke could be induction of rapid defibrinogenation by the viper venom ancrod (Bell et al., 1968). Defibrinogenation produces anticoagulation by depleting the substrate needed for thrombus formation; additionally, reduction of fibrinogen also decreases blood viscosity, resulting in improved organ perfusion and the products of defibrinogenation enhance local thrombolysis by stimulating endogenous plasminogen activators (Pollak et al., 1990). After some experience has been obtained with this compound in reperfusion therapy for various clinical conditions, e.g., peripheral vascular disease, deep vein thrombosis and central retinal venous thrombosis ancrod was applied in small randomized studies (Hossmann et al., 1983; Olinger et al., 1988) and a larger multicenter trial (The Ancrod Stroke Study Investigators, 1994). These studies suggested that ancrod was both safe and beneficial in stroke patients; the multicenter trial demonstrated even a significant benefit in neurological function measured by the Scandinavian Stroke Scale and a trend on the Barthel Index of functional capability and for mortality.

In a large randomized, parallel group, double-blind, placebo-controlled multicenter trial (Sherman et al., 2000) this beneficial effect of intravenous ancrod for treatment of acute ischemic stroke was confirmed. A total of 500 patients with acute or progressing ischemic neurological deficit were enrolled and included in the intention-to-treat-analysis. Patients randomly received ancrod (n = 248) or placebo (n = 252) as a continuous 72h intravenous infusion beginning within 3h of stroke onset, followed by 1h infusion at 96 and 120h. This regimen was designed to decrease plasma fibrinogen levels to 1.18–2.03 µmol/l. Favorable outcome, defined as survival to day 90 with a Barthel Index of 95 or more, was achieved by more patients in the ancrod group (42.2%) than in the placebo group (34.4%, P = 0.04). Mortality was not different between the groups (25.4% for ancrod, 23% for placebo) and the proportion of severely disabled patients was less in the ancrod group than in the placebo group (11.8% vs. 19.8%, P = 0.01). Symptomatic intracranial hemorrhages were insignificantly (5.2% vs. 2.0%, P = 0.06) and asymptomatic hemorrhages were significantly increased in the ancrod group (19.0% vs. 10.7%, P = 0.01). These beneficial effects of ancrod, however, could not be duplicated in an European multicenter trial (Orgogozo et al., 2000) which was under powered to significantly demonstrate its efficacy, and ancrod has not been approved yet for treatment of acute stroke.

Hemodilution and volume expansion

Experimental animal and human studies have demonstrated that hemodilution significantly increases regional blood flow in normal and hypoperfused brain tissue (Heiss et al., 1972). As the level of residual blood flow is a major determinant of the extent of the final infarct, hemodilution has been expected to improve functional outcome following focal cerebral ischemia and therefore was widely applied in patients with stroke (Gottstein, 1984). However, a number of controlled trials summarized in a meta-analysis (Asplund, 1991) failed to prove any clinical benefit from this treatment. Inclusion criteria of these studies permitted 12–48h for entry into treatment regimens and pre-existing hypovolemia as well as insufficient fluid application may have counteracted a potential benefit of hemodilution. Additionally, low molecular weight dextran used in most of these studies is not the best choice for hemodilution, since it even might increase plasma viscosity, may aggravate brain edema and conveys the risk of anaphylactic reactions. A newly developed hydroxyethyl starch (HES) solution with a mean molecular weight of 130 ± 20kD and a molar substitution of 0.4 might be better suited since it is rapidly metabolized and eliminated via the kidneys. In a double blind, placebo controlled, randomized multicenter trial a 10% solution of HES 130/0.4 was tested versus 0.9% saline solution in 106 patients with acute stroke (Rudolf et

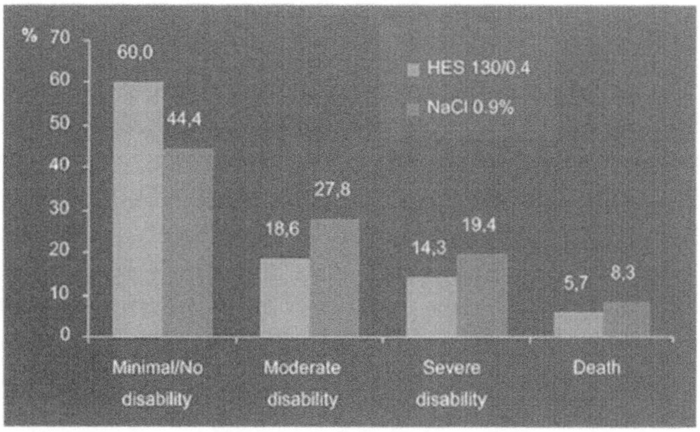

Fig. 3. Modified Rankin Scale scores 3 months after the stroke for the HES 130/0.4 (n = 70) and the NaCl 0.9% (n = 36) groups. The trend to better outcome for the HES group did not reach statistical significance

al., 2002). HES or placebo was initiated within 6h of symptom onset and repeated every 8h on days 1–3 and every 24h on days 4–7. In this phase II safety study there was no significant difference between the groups with regard to the incidence of specific adverse events (cardiovascular events, bleeding complications, allergic reactions) assessed over days 1–30 or for mortality over days 1–8. In addition, despite the study was not powered to prove efficacy, a trend towards a better functional outcome with HES therapy was observed in global tests. In the HES group 7.4% more patients than in the placebo group reached the minimal/no disability group on the Rankin Scale (Fig. 3). If confirmed in a larger trial this trend would be comparable to the effect of systemic rt-PA rendering hemodilution a promising alternative to thrombolysis applicable to a larger group of stroke patients.

Anticoagulants and antiplatelet therapy

Immediate anticoagulant therapy, — full or low-dose unfractionated heparin, low-molecular-weight heparins, heparinoids, oral anticoagulants and thrombin inhibitors — in patients with acute ischemic stroke is not associated with net short- or long-term benefit (Gubitz et al., 2001a). Antiplatelet therapy with 160–300 mg aspirin daily and started within 48 h of onset of ischemic stroke reduces the risk of early recurrent stroke without a major risk of early hemorrhagic complications and improves long-term outcome (Gubitz et al., 2001b). Both strategies cannot be considered acute interventions with the pathophysiologic events leading to ischemic brain damage, but represent means for early secondary prevention of recurrent stroke.

Neuroprotection

In acute ischemic stroke the damage is initiated by hypoperfusion with depletion of oxygen and energy supply to the tissue. A cascade of neurotoxicity follows with release of glutamate, glycine, free radicals, nitric oxide, and other mediators of cell damage, leading to disturbance of ionic equilibrium with calcium influx into the cells and osmotic swelling as well as inflammatory changes and induction of apoptotic mechanisms (Barone and Feuerstein, 1999; Dirnagl et al., 1999; Schulz et al., 1999). While many of the mechanisms contributing to ischemic cell damage have been described during the last years, no pharmacologic agent has yet shown efficacy in the human's brain ischemic cascade once it starts to spread (Plum, 2001). In a recent review De Keyser et al. (1999) described 22 completed phase 3 trials of neuroprotective pharmacologic drugs, all of which failed. This result, which was also reported in the recent glycine antagonist trials (Lees et al., 2000; Sacco et al., 2001), is disappointing since these strategies had definite benefits in animal models decreasing the final infarcts by up to 50% compared to untreated controls (Barinaga, 1998; Hickenbottom and Grotta, 1998). In addition, some of the drugs were shown to increase blood flow to the ischemic territory and to reduce the penumbra zone with an eventual effect on the size of the final infarct (review in Hakim, 1989; Heiss, 2000). The failure to translate results from animal models to humans probably has many causes (De Keyser et al., 1999; Liebeskind and Kasner, 2001), as inconsequences in trial design — e.g., initiation of treatment beyond the window of opportunity and/or with inadequate dosage —, limitations of the current drug development process to animal models which do not reflect the pathophysiological condition of human stroke, and the heterogeneity of the stroke population, where a specified drug action to correct a particular pathophysiologic aberration can only be effective in a small number of individuals. Recently it was even argued that most strategies applied up to now were targeted against ineffective mechanisms (Lee et al., 1999). In the future, therefore, neuroprotective trials must be conducted on patients' populations selected carefully with respect to type and site of ischemia and to the pathophysiological disturbance that the tested compound was designed to treat. Functional imaging modalities, as DW- and PW-MRI, PET or SPECT might help to identify more rationally appropriate candidates and additionally could be used as surrogate measures of efficacy for neuroprotective therapies.

Since the primary target of neuroprotective treatment is rather small — only a rather small portion of the final infarct is initially outside the critically hypoperfused area (Heiss et al., 2001b) — we should not expect that any single drug that interferes with a specific event in the ischemic cascade will have a large clinical impact. The effects especially when studied in heterogenous groups of patients, might not be measurable with the crude clinical outcome measures that are currently used. Instead of continuing with single drug trials it might be more rewarding to explore treatments using a combination of reperfusion with neuroprotection and a cocktail of carefully selected neuroprotective drugs (De Keyser et al., 1999; Kaste, 2001).

General management

Specific ischemic stroke treatment with thrombolytics, the only drugs that have demonstrated efficacy in reducing morbidity associated with stroke, is applicable only to a very small number of acute stroke patients (1–6% of all stroke victims, Chiu et al., 1998). Thrombolysis, therefore, has little influence on stroke mortality and morbidity in the general population. This is due, in part, to the strict time window in which the drug may be administered and also to the reluctance of physicians to administer a drug that is potentially harmful. That means, that the management of acute stroke victims and the education of treating physicians must be improved. In keeping with these assumptions the management of patients suffering acute stroke has been organized in many communities involving the emergency system, the general practitioners and internists, the medical departments in the community hospitals and the neurological departments as centers of the dedicated network. Within this operational network stroke units and multidisciplinary teams that deliver the stroke service play an important role. Organized stroke care can apply various models, which all share the following characteristics: a staff specialized in stroke, a coordinated multidisciplinary team, and an accepted protocol for diagnosis, specific treatment and interventions for adverse physiological changes. Stroke units are different with respect to their composition and to the service they provide: Specially organized stroke units can be a ward or a team that exclusively manages stroke patients (a dedicated stroke unit) or a ward or team that provides a general disability service (a mixed assessment or rehabilitation unit) (Stroke Unit Trialists' Collaboration, 2001). This Cochrane Review has documented that irrespective of the type of model used stroke patients who receive organized in patient care in a stroke unit are more likely to be alive (odd ratio 0.83), independent (OR 0.75), and living at home (OR 0.77) one year after the stroke. The apparent benefits are not restricted to any particular sub-groups of patients; no systematic increase was observed in the length of inpatient stay. Within 5 years of stroke the relative risk of death has been reduced by 40% in the patients treated in a stroke unit (Jorgensen et al., 1999), and this result has been confirmed 10 years after the initial stroke (Indredavik et al., 1999) (Table 1). The more favorable outcome was related to early mobilization and rehabilitation of patients, the stabiliza-

Table 1. Effect of stroke unit on mortality

	Standard	Stroke unit	Effect
1 month	23%	14%	−9%
6 months	31%	24%	−7%
1 year	37%	31%	−6%
5 years	71%	59%	−12%
10 years	87%	76%	−11%
Number needed to treat to avoid 1 death:	10		

Stroke (1998) 29: 58–62; Stroke (1997) 28: 1861–1866; Stroke (1999) 30: 1524–1527

Table 2. Comparative effectiveness of acute treatment strategies

Intervention	RRR	ARR	NNT	Target Population	Adverse Outcomes Avoided
Stroke Unit	9%	5.6%	18	80%	107
Aspirin	3%	1.2%	83	80%	23
Thrombolysis (rtPA)	17%	12%	8	5%	14

◆ Assumes population of 1,000,000 with 2,400 first and recurrent strokes annually
◆ Thrombolysis is IV rtPA 0–3 h after onset

Adapted from Hankey and Warlow (1999; Lancet 354: 1457–1463)

tion of blood pressure and the reduction of medical complications. With a dedicated stroke unit the outcome could be further improved compared to the outcome obtained with a stroke team (OR 0.46) and compared to the outcome with conventional treatment at home (OR 0.59) (Kalra et al., 2000). Especially careful monitoring of blood pressure (Wahlgren et al., 1994) and control of blood glucose level (Weir et al., 1997) have a significant impact on outcome after stroke. Overall, treatment in specialized stroke units is the most successful and most cost effective strategy to improve outcome after ischemic stroke (number needed to treat to prevent one additional death 24, to prevent death or dependency 18) and therefore, the widespread implementation of stroke units in urban and rural settings must be the priority of health programs in the fight against stroke. With the broad applicability and the wide distribution of stroke units the impact of this measure to improve the outcome after stroke is very high (Table 2).

Special interventions in malignant infarctions

Some patients with acute infarction of most of the middle cerebral artery territory or of most of the hemisphere develop massive edema leading to significant midline shift, compression of the basal cisterna and finally to uncal herniation with brain stem dysfunction. The critical condition usually is reached with intracerebral pressure increased above 30 mmHg 2 to 5 days after the stroke (Hacke et al., 1996). In this malignant MCA infarction standard antiedema treatment often fails, mortality is high (80%) and surviving patients are usually severely disabled. The development of malignant brain infarction can be predicted from early CT findings in patients with MCA occlusion (von Kummer et al., 1994): a hypodensity covering more than 50% of the MCA territory or local brain swelling (effacement of sulci, compression of the lateral ventricle) are indicators of bad prognosis; large (>50%) or total hypodensity in the MCA territory predicted fatal outcome in 85% with a high specificity (94%) but moderate sensitivity (64%). Treatment of brain edema is therefore an important interventional strategy to prevent or reduce elevated intracranial pressure and its consequences.

Osmotherapy

Infusion of hyperosmolar solutions can extract water from brain tissue and therefore reduce the volume even of normal brain. The goal of osmotherapy is to increase serum osmolarity for a period sufficient to reduce the water content of the brain, but without causing intravascular fluid overload which may evoke rebound phenomena. Glycerol in 10% solutions have been used successfully (Mathew et al., 1972), but results have been controversial (Restrepo and Silverman, 2001), and large scale controlled trials are missing. In a systemic review including 11 randomized trials in patients with definite probable ischemic stroke (Righetti et al., 2000) glycerol was associated with a significant reduction in the odds of death during the scheduled treatment period (OR 0.65, 95% CI 0.44–0.97) although this favorable outcome could not be detected at the end of the scheduled follow-up period (OR 0.98).

Mannitol (20% solutions) holds an eminent position in the limited instrumentarium of neurological critical care and is preferred for more severe cases of stroke, despite well designed studies addressing its efficiency in stroke are missing (Bereczki et al., 2000). It has a higher risk of fluid overloads and should be applied as short infusions every 4h if glycerol fails to control elevated ICP. The other measures used to reduce elevated intracranial pressure in neurosurgical conditions, e.g. hyperventilation, have not been effective in ischemic stroke (Steiner et al., 2001).

Decompressive surgery

The rationale for decompressive surgery is to allow expansion of edematous tissue away from the critical structures in the diencephalon and the mesencephalon, to reduce intracerebral pressure in order to preserve sufficient perfusion pressure and to prevent further compression of collateral vessels. These factors may help to stabilize perfusion in areas surrounding infarcted regions, thereby preventing further tissue necrosis. Case series impressively show a dramatic reduction of mortality in patients with both, cerebellar and hemispheric space-occupying infarctions, if decompressive surgery is performed early in the course. The Heidelberg trials are the only prospectively designed trials and include data from a non-randomized control group (Steiner et al., 2001). Without surgery 76% of patients with space-occupying hemispheric infarction died from herniation despite maximal conservative treatment. The mortality in the surgically treated group (n = 32) was significantly lower (32%), with 14 of the surviving patients (21) independent or mildly to moderately disabled, and 80% reaching a Barthel Index of 60 or above. When surgical intervention time was reduced from an average of 39h after stroke to 21h in the second part of this study (n = 31) mortality was further reduced to 16% and 17 patients recovered to an independent or moderately disabled state.

This experience indicates the efficacy of decompressive surgery for improving outcome after malignant brain infarction, but also stresses the importance of patient selection and timing of intervention. Studies are now underway to evaluate the role of invasive monitoring (microdialysis of chemical substrates, intracranial pressure, O_2 tissue saturation) and of functional imaging (DW- and PW-MRI, $H_2{}^{15}O$ and FMZ-PET) for the identification of stroke patients which may benefit from decompressive surgery (Schneweis et al., 2001; Steiner et al., 2001).

Hypothermia

Moderate hypothermia (33–36°C) has been shown to reduce secondary brain injury and infarction size and to improve neurologic outcome in animal models of focal and global ischemia (Busto et al., 1989; Karibe et al., 1994). In the first clinical trial on the use of moderate hypothermia in severe MCA infarction, initiated within 14h and maintained over 72h, mortality was reduced to 44% and the survivors reached a favorable outcome (Schwab et al., 1998). The rewarming period, however, was critical leading to secondary rises of intracranial pressure. Based on these observations a multicenter trial is planned in which direct brain cooling devices (helmets, infusions) should reach the predefined temperatures more rapidly and should limit systemic side effects.

Conclusions

Acute interventions based on pathophysiological concepts of the ischemic brain damage have replaced the nihilistic approach to therapy of acute ischemic stroke. However, since the only approved treatment — thrombolysis within a rather short time window — is limited to a small portion of the stroke population (~5%) further efforts are necessary to develop strategies from which more stroke victims can benefit and which can improve the outcome in severe conditions.

References

Adams HPJr, Brott TG, Furlan AJ, Gomez CR, Grotta J, Helgason CM, Kwiatkowski T, Lyden PD, Marler JR, Torner J, Feinberg W, Mayberg M, Thies W (1996) Guidelines for thrombolytic therapy for acute stroke: a supplement to the guidelines for the management of patients with acute ischemic stroke. A statement for healthcare professionals from a special writing group of the Stroke Council, American Heart Association. Ciculation 94: 1167–1174

Albers GW (1999) Expanding the window for thrombolytic therapy in acute stroke. The potential role of acute MRI for patient selection. Stroke 30: 2230–2237

Albers GW, Bates VE, Clark WM, Bell R, Verro P, Hamilton SA (2000) Intravenous tissue-type plasminogen activator for treatment of acute stroke: the Standard Treatment with Alteplase to Reverse Stroke (STARS) study. JAMA 283: 1145–1150

Asplund K (1991) Hemodilution in acute stroke. Cerebrovasc Dis [Suppl]: 129–138

Astrup J, Siesjö BK, Symon L (1981) Thresholds in cerebral ischemia — the ischemic penumbra. Stroke 12: 723–725

Barinaga M (1998) Stroke-damaged neurons may commit cellular suicide. Science 281: 1302–1303

Baron JC, Bousser MG, Rey A, Guillard A, Comar D, Castaigne P (1981) Reversal of focal "misery-perfusion syndrome" by extra-intracranial arterial bypass in hemodynamic cerebral ischemia. A case study with ^{15}O positron emission tomography. Stroke 12: 454–459

Barone FC, Feuerstein GZ (1999) Inflammatory mediators and stroke: new opportunities for novel therapeutics. J Cereb Blood Flow Metab 19: 819–834

Bell WR, Pitney WR, Goodwin JF (1968) Therapeutic defibrination in the treatment of thrombotic disease. Lancet i: 490–493

Bereczki D, Lui M, do Prado GF, Fekete I (2000) A systematic review of mannitol therapy for acute ischemic stroke and cerebral parenchymal hemorrhage. Stroke 31: 2722

Busto R, Dietrich WD, Globus MY, Ginsberg MD (1989) Postischemic moderate hypothermia inhibits CA1 hippocampal ischemic neuronal injury. Neurosci Lett 101: 299–304

Chapman KM, Woolfenden AR, Graeb D, Johnston DC, Beckman J, Schulzer M, Teal PA (2000) Intravenous tissue plasminogen activator for acute ischemic stroke: a Canadian hospital's experience. Stroke 31: 2920–2924

Chiu D, Krieger D, Villar-Cordova C, Kasner SE, Morgenstern LB, Bratina PL, Yatsu FM, Grotta JC (1998) Intravenous tissue plasminogen activator for acute ischemic stroke. Feasibility, safety, and efficacy in the first year of clinical practice. Stroke 29: 18–22

Davenport J, Hanson SK, Altafullah IM, Anderson DC, Brauer DJ, Brown RD, Ramirez-Lassepas M (2000) tPA: A rural network experience. Stroke 31: 1457

De Keyser J, Sulter G, Luiten PG (1999) Clinical trials with neuroprotective drugs in acute ischaemic stroke: are we doing the right thing? TINS-Trends Neurosci 22: 535–540

del Zoppo GJ, Poeck K, Pessin MS, Wolpert SM, Furlan AJ, Ferbert A, Alberts MJ, Zivin JA, Wechsler L, Busse O, Greenlee R, Brass L, Mohr JP, Feldmann E, Hacke W, Kase CS, Biller J, Gress D, Otis SM (1992) Recombinant tissue plasminogen activator in acute thrombotic and embolic stroke. Ann Neurol 32: 78–86

Dirnagl U, Iadecola C, Moskowitz MA (1999) Pathobiology of ischaemic stroke: an integrated view. TINS-Trends Neurosci 22: 391–397

Fieschi C, Argentino C, Lenzi GL, Sacchetti ML, Toni D, Bozzao L (1989) Clinical and instrumental evaluation of patients with ischemic stroke within the first six hours. J Neurol Sci 91: 311–322

Fisher M, Albers GW (1999) Applications of diffusion-perfusion magnetic resonance imaging in acute ischemic stroke. Neurology 52: 1750–1756

Furlan A, Higashida R, Wechsler L, Gent M, Rowley H, Kase C, Pessin M, Ahuja A, Callahan F, Clark WM, Silver F, Rivera F (1999) Intra-arterial prourokinase for acute ischemic stroke. The PROACT II study: a randomized controlled trial. JAMA-J Am Med Assoc 282: 2003–2011

Gottstein U (1984) Hemodilution: therapy in acute ischemic stroke. In: Bes A, Braquet P, Paoletti R, Siesjö BK (eds) Cerebral ischemia. Elsevier Science Publishers B.V., Amsterdam, pp 311–324

Grond M, Stenzel C, Schmülling S, Rudolf J, Neveling M, Lechleuthner A, Schneweis S, Heiss W-D (1998) Early intravenous thrombolysis for acute ischemic stroke in a community-based approach. Stroke 29: 1544–1549

Grotta J (1994) The current status of neuronal protective therapy: why have all neuronal protective drugs worked in animals but none so far in stroke patients? Cerebrovasc Dis 4: 115–120

Grotta JC, Alexandrov AV (1998) tPA-associated reperfusion after acute stroke demonstrated by SPECT. Stroke 29: 429–432

Gubitz G, Counsell C, Sandercock P, Signorini D (2001a) Anticoagulants for acute ischaemic stroke (Cochrane Review). The Cochrane Library 3

Gubitz G, Sandercock P, Counsell C (2001b) Antiplatelet therapy for acute ischaemic stroke (Cochrane Review). The Cochrane Library 3

Hacke W, Kaste M, Fieschi C, Toni D, Lesaffre E, von Kummer R, Boysen G, Bluhmki E, Höxter G, Mahagne MH, Hennerici M (1995) Intravenous thrombolysis with recombinant tissue plasminogen activator for acute hemispheric stroke. The European Cooperative Acute Stroke Study (ECASS). JAMA-J Am Med Assoc 274: 1017–1025

Hacke W, Schwab S, Horn M, Spranger M, De Georgia M, von Kummer R (1996) "Malignant" middle cerebral artery territory infarction: clinical course and prognostic signs. Arch Neurol 53: 309–315

Hacke W, Kaste M, Fieschi C, von Kummer R, Davalos A, Meier D, Larrue V, Bluhmki E, Davis S, Donnan G, Schneider D, Diez-Tejedor E, Trouillas P (1998) Randomised double-blind placebo-controlled trial of thrombolytic therapy with intravenous alteplase in acute ischemic stroke (ECASS II). Lancet 352: 1245–1251

Hacke W, Brott T, Caplan L, Meier D, Fieschi C, von Kummer R, Donnan G, Heiss W-D, Wahlgren NG, Spranger M, Boysen G, Marler JR (1999) Thrombolysis in acute ischemic stroke: controlled trials and clinical experience. Neurology 53:S3–14

Hakim AM (1989) Hemodynamic and metabolic studies in stroke. Semin Neurol 9: 286–292

Hakim AM, Pokrupa RP, Villanueva J, Diksic M, Evans AC, Thompson CJ, Meyer E, Yamamoto YL, Feindel WH (1987) The effect of spontaneous reperfusion on metabolic function in early human cerebral infarcts. Ann Neurol 21: 279–289

Heiss W-D (2000) Ischemic penumbra: evidence from functional imaging in man. J Cereb Blood Flow Metab 20: 1276–1293

Heiss W-D, Graf R (1994) The ischemic penumbra. Curr Opin Neurol 7: 11–19

Heiss W-D, Prosenz P, Tschabitscher H, Lasek C, Herles HJ (1972) Effect of low molecular dextran on total cerebral blood flow and on regional flow within ischemic brain lesions. Eur Neurol 8: 129–133

Heiss W-D, Grond M, Thiel A, von Stockhausen HM, Rudolf J, Ghaemi M, Löttgen J, Stenzel C, Pawlik G (1998) Tissue at risk of infarction rescued by early reperfusion: a positron emission tomography study in systemic recombinant tissue plasminogen activator thrombolysis of acute stroke. J Cereb Blood Flow Metab 18: 1298–1307

Heiss W-D, Thiel A, Grond M, Graf R (1999) Which targets are relevant for therapy of acute ischemic stroke? Stroke 30: 1486–1489

Heiss W-D, Kracht L, Grond M, Rudolf J, Bauer B, Wienhard K, Pawlik G (2000) Early [^{11}C]Flumazenil/H_2O positron emission tomography predicts irreversible ischemic cortical damage in stroke patients receiving acute thrombolytic therapy. Stroke 31: 366–369

Heiss W-D, Graf R, Wienhard K (2001a) Relevance of experimental ischemia in cats for stroke management: a comparative reevaluation. Cerebrovasc Dis 11: 73–81

Heiss W-D, Kracht LW, Thiel A, Grond M, Pawlik G (2001b) Penumbral probability thresholds of cortical flumazenil binding and blood flow predicting tissue outcome in patients with cerebral ischaemia. Brain 124: 20–29

Hickenbottom SL, Grotta J (1998) Neuroprotective therapy. Semin Neurol 18: 485–492

Hossmann K-A (1994) Viability thresholds and the penumbra of focal ischemia. Ann Neurol 36: 557–565

Hossmann V, Heiss W-D, Bewermeyer H, Wiedemann G (1983) Controlled trial of ancrod in ischemic stroke. Arch Neurol 40: 803–808

Indredavik B, Bakke F, Slordahl SA, Rokseth R, Haheim LL (1999) Stroke unit treatment. 10-Year follow-up. Stroke 30: 1524–1527

Jansen O, Schellinger P, Fiebach J, Hacke W, Sartor K (1999) Early recanalisation in acute ischaemic stroke saves tissue at risk defined by MRI. Lancet 353: 2036–2037

Jorgensen HS, Kammersgaard LP, Nakayama H, Raaschou HO, Larsen K, Hubbe P, Olsen TS (1999) Treatment and rehabilitation on a stroke unit improves 5-year survival. A community-based study. Stroke 30: 930–933

Kalra L, Evans A, Perez I, Knapp M, Donaldson N, Swift CG (2000) Alternative strategies for stroke care: a prospective randomised controlled trial. Lancet 356: 894–899

Karibe H, Chen J, Zarow GJ, Graham SH, Weinstein PR (1994) Delayed induction of mild hypothermia to reduce infarct volume after temporary middle cerebral artery occlusion in rats. J Neurosurg 80: 112–119

Kaste M (2001) Thrombolysis in ischaemic stroke — present and future: role of combined therapy. Cerebrovasc Dis 11 [Suppl 1]: 55–59

Katzan IL, Furlan AJ, Lloyd LE, Frank JI, Harper DL, Hinchey JA, Hammel JP, Qu A, Sila CA (2000) Use of tissue-type plasminogen activator for acute ischemic stroke: the Cleveland area experience. JAMA 283: 1151–1158

Kidwell CS, Saver JL, Mattiello J, Starkman S, Vinuela F, Duckwiler G, Gobin YP, Jahan R, Vespa P, Kalafut M, Alger JR (2000) Thrombolytic reversal of acute human cerebral ischemic injury shown by diffusion/perfusion magnetic resonance imaging. Ann Neurol 47: 462–469

Klotz E, König M (1999) Perfusion measurements of the brain: using dynamic CT for the quantitative assessment of cerebral ischemia in acute stroke. Eur J Radiol 30: 170–184

Koroshetz WJ, Gonzales RG (1999) Imaging stroke in progress: magnetic resonance advances but computed tomography is poised for counterattack. Ann Neurol 46: 556–558

Kwiatkowski TG, Libman RB, Frankel M, Tilley BC, Morgenstern LB, Lu M, Broderick JP, Lewandowski CA, Marler JR, Levine SR, Brott T (1999) Effects of tissue plasminogen activator for acute ischemic stroke at one year. National Institute of Neurological Disorders and Stroke Recombinant Tissue Plasminogen Activator Stroke Study Group. N Engl J Med 340: 1781–1787

Lee JM, Zipfel GJ, Choi DW (1999) The changing landscape of ischaemic brain injury mechanisms. Nature 399:A7–A14

Lees KR, Asplund K, Carolei A, Davis SM, Diener HC, Kaste M, Orgogozo J-M, Whitehead J (2000) Glycine antagonist (gavestinel) in neuroprotection (GAIN International) in patients with acute stroke: a randomised controlled trial. GAIN International Investigators. Lancet 355: 1949–1954

Liebeskind DS, Kasner SE (2001) Neuroprotection for ischaemic stroke: an unattainable goal? CNS Drugs 15: 165–174

Marks MP, Tong DC, Beaulieu C, Albers GW, de Crespigny A, Moseley ME (1999) Evaluation of early reperfusion and IV tPA therapy using diffusion- and perfusion-weighted MRI. Neurology 52: 1792–1798

Mathew NT, Meyer JS, Rivera VM, Charney JZ, Hartmann A (1972) Double-blind evaluation of glycerol treatment in acute cerebral infarction. Lancet ii: 1327–1329

Olinger CP, Brott TG, Barsan WG, Hedges JR, Glas-Greenwalt P, Pollak VE, Spilker J, Eberle R (1988) Use of ancrod in acute or progressing ischemic cerebral infarction. Ann Emerg Med 17: 1208–1209

Orgogozo JM, Verstraete M, Kay R, Hennerici M, Lenzi GL (2000) Outcomes of ancrod in acute ischemic stroke. Independent Data and Safety Monitoring Board for ESTAT. Steering Committee for ESTAT. European Stroke Treatment with Ancrod Trial. JAMA 284: 1926–1927

Plum F (2001) Neuroprotection in acute ischemic stroke. JAMA 285: 1760–1761

Pollak VE, Glas-Greenwalt P, Olinger CP, Wadhwa NK, Myre SA (1990) Ancrod causes rapid thrombolysis in patients with acute stroke. Am J Med Sci 299: 319–325

Restrepo L, Silverman IE (2001) Osmotherapy: a call to arms. Stroke 32: 811–812

Righetti E, Celani MG, Cantisani T, Sterzi R, Boysen G, Ricci S (2000) Glycerol for acute stroke (Cochrane Review). The Cochrane Library 3

Rubin G, Firlik AD, Pindzola RR, Levy EI, Yonas H (1999) The effect of reperfusion therapy on cerebral blood flow in acute stroke. J Stroke Cerebrovasc Dis 8: 1–9

Rudolf J, et al (2002) Hydroxyethyl starch for hypervolemic hemodilution in patients with acute ischemic stroke — a randomized, placebo-controlled phase II safety study. Cerebrovasc Dis 14: 33–41

Ryu YH, Chung TS, Yoon PH, Kim DI, Lee JD, Lee BI, Suh JH (1999) Evaluation of reperfusion and recovery of brain function before and after intracarotid arterial urokinase therapy in acute cerebral infarction with brain SPECT. Clin Nucl Med 24: 566–571

Sacco RL, DeRosa JT, Haley EC, Jr, Levin B, Ordronneau P, Phillips SJ, Rundek T, Snipes RG, Thompson JL (2001) Glycine antagonist in neuroprotection for patients with acute stroke: GAIN Americas: a randomized controlled trial. JAMA 285: 1719–1728

Sasaki O, Takeuchi S, Koizumi T, Koike T, Tanaka R (1996) Complete recanalization via fibrinolytic therapy can reduce the number of ischemic territories that progress to infarction. Am J Neuroradiol 17: 1661–1668

Saver JL, Johnston KC, Homer D, Wityk R, Koroshetz W, Truskowski LL, Haley EC (1999) Infarct volume as a surrogate or auxiliary outcome measure in ischemic stroke clinical trials. The RANTTAS Investigators. Stroke 30: 293–298

Schellinger PD, Jansen O, Fiebach JB, Heiland S, Steiner T, Schwab S, Pohlers O, Ryssel H, Sartor K, Hacke W (2000) Monitoring intravenous recombinant tissue plasminogen activator thrombolysis for acute ischemic stroke with diffusion and perfusion MRI. Stroke 31: 1318–1328

Schmülling S, Grond M, Rudolf J, Heiss W-D (2000) One-year follow-up in acute stroke patients treated with rtPA in clinical routine. Stroke 31: 1552–1554

Schneweis S, Grond M, Staub F, Brinker G, Neveling M, Dohmen C, Graf R, Heiss W-D (2001) Predictive value of neurochemical monitoring in large middle cerebral artery infarction. Stroke 32: 1863–1867

Schulz JB, Weller M, Moskowitz MA (1999) Caspases as treatment targets in stroke and neurodegenerative diseases. Ann Neurol 45: 421–429

Schwab S, Schwarz S, Spranger M, Keller E, Bertram M, Hacke W (1998) Moderate hypothermia in the treatment of patients with severe middle cerebral artery infarction. Stroke 29: 2461–2466

Segal AZ, Lev MH, Schwamm HL, Jeffery F, Jonathan R, Putman CM, Budzik RF, Hunter GJ, Rordorf G, Buonanno F, Koroshetz W, Gonzalez G (1999) CT-perfusion imaging in acute stroke with MCA stem occlusion: prediciting outcome after intra-arterial (IA) thrombolysis. Stroke 30: 248

Sherman DG, Atkinson RP, Chippendale T, Levin KA, Ng K, Futrell N, Hsu CY, Levy DE, for the STAT Participants (2000) Intravenous ancrod for treatment of acute ischemic stroke. The STAT study: a randomized controlled trial. JAMA-J Am Med Assoc 283: 2395–2403

Steiner T, Ringleb P, Hacke W (2001) Treatment options for large hemispheric stroke. Neurology 57 [Suppl 2]: S61–S68

Stroke Unit Trialists' Collaboration (2001) Organised inpatient (stroke unit) care for stroke (Cochrane Review). The Cochrane Library 3

Tanne D, Demchuk AM, Kasner SE, Grond M, Hanson SK, Hamilton S, Buchan AM, Wang DZ, Wechsler LR, Zweifler RM, Levine SR (2000) A large multinational investigation to predict t-PA related symptomatic ICH in patients with acute ischemic stroke. Stroke 30: 248

The Ancrod Stroke Study Investigators (1994) Ancrod for the treatment of acute ischemic brain infarction. Stroke 25: 1755–1759

The European Ad Hoc Consensus Group (1996) European strategies for early internention in stroke. Cerebrovasc Dis 6: 315–324

The NINDS rt-PA Stroke Study Group (1995) Tissue plasminogen activator for acute ischemic stroke. N Engl J Med 333: 1581–1587

Trouillas P, Nighoghossian N, Derex L, Adeleine P, Honnorat J, Neuschwander P, Riche G, Getenet JC, Li W, Froment JC, Turjman F, Malicier D, Fournier G, Gabry AL,

Ledoux X, Berthezene Y, Ffrench P, Dechavanne M (1998) Thrombolysis with intravenous rtPA in a series of 100 cases of acute carotid territory stroke: determination of etiological, topographic, and radiological outcome factors. Stroke 29: 2529–2540

Ueda T, Sakaki S, Yuh WTC, Nochide I, Ohta S (1999) Outcome in acute stroke with successful intra-arterial thrombolysis and predictive value of initial single-photon emission-computed tomography. J Cereb Blood Flow Metab 19: 99–108

von Kummer R, Meyding-Lamade U, Forsting M, Rosin L, Rieke K, Hacke W, Sartor K (1994) Sensitivity and prognostic value of early CT in occlusion of the middle cerebral artery trunk. AJNR Am J Neuroradiol 15: 9–15

Wahlgren NG, Macmahon DG, De Keyser J, Indredavik B, Ryman T (1994) Intravenous nimodipine West-European Stroke Trial (INWEST) of nimodipine in the treatment of acute ischaemic stroke. Cerebrovasc Dis 4: 204–210

Wang DZ, Rose JA, Honings DS, Garwacki DJ, Milbrandt JC (2000) Treating acute stroke patients with intravenous tPA. The OSF stroke network experience. Stroke 31: 77–81

Wardlaw JM, Warlow CP, Counsell C (1997) Systematic review of evidence on thrombolytic therapy for acute ischemic stroke. Lancet 350: 607–614

Wardlaw JM, Del Zoppo G, Yamaguchi T (2000) Thrombolysis versus control in acute ischemic stroke (Cochrane Review). Cochrane Library 3

Weir CJ, Murray GD, Dyker AG, Lees KR (1997) Is hyperglycaemia an independent predictor of poor outcome after acute stroke? Results of a long-term follow up study. BMJ 314: 1303–1306

Author's address: Prof. Dr. W.-D. Heiss, Max-Planck-Institut für neurologische Forschung, Gleueler Strasse 50, D-50931 Köln, Federal Republic of Germany, e-mail: wdh@pet.mpin-koeln.mpg.de

J Neural Transm (2002) [Suppl] 63: 59–73

Rehabilitation approaches to stroke

F. Aichner, C. Adelwöhrer, and **H.-P. Haring**

Department of Neurology, Wagner-Jauregg Hospital, Linz, Teaching Hospital, University Innsbruck, Linz, Austria

Summary. This article describes the state of the science in stroke rehabilitation dealing with three main topics:

(1) General approach to stroke rehabilitation (stroke services and stroke units),
(2) Neurophysiological and pharmacological interventions (facilitation of brain repair mechanisms) and
(3) Experimental approaches (neuronal transplantation)

Stroke rehabilitation is an active process beginning during acute hospitalisation, progressing to a systematic program of rehabilitation services and continuing after the individual returns to the community. There is world-wide consensus that stroke patients should be treated at specialised stroke unit with specially trained medical and nursing staff, co-ordinated multidisciplinary rehabilitation and education programs for patients and their families. Stroke Unit has been shown to be associated with a long-term reduction of death and of the combined poor outcomes of death and dependency, independent of patients age, sex, or variations in stroke unit organisations. No study has clearly shown to what extent the beneficial effect is due to specific rehabilitation strategies.

New imaging studies in stroke patients indicate altered post stroke activation patterns, which suggest some functional reorganisation. Reorganisation may be the principle process responsible for recovery after stroke. It is assumed that different post ischaemic interventions like physiotherapy, occupational therapy, speech therapy, electrical stimulation, etc. facilitates such changes. Scientific evidence demonstrating the values of specific rehabilitation interventions after stroke is limited. Comparisons between different methods in current use have so far mostly failed to show that any particular physiotherapy, occupational therapy, speech therapy or stroke rehabilitation strategy is superior to another. Clinical data are strongly in favour of early mobilisation and training.

Pharmacological interventions in animals revealed that norepinephrine, amphetamine and other alpha-adrenergic stimulating drugs can enhance motor performance after unilateral ablation of the sensory motor cortex. The clinical data in humans are rather contradictory.

Neural grafting and neurogenesis are new potential modes of stroke therapy. Neural grafting enhanced functional outcome and reduced thalamic atrophy in rats only when combined with housing in enriched environments. Recent studies have shown that stem cells can differentiate to neurons in the adult human dentate gyrus in vivo.

Introduction

Stroke is both common and serious. It has been estimated that in 1990 stroke caused 4,4 million deaths world wide. Within most western countries a typical district of 250,000 people might expect more than 500 new strokes per year, of whom a half will have died or remain physically dependent one year later. Because so many survivors remain disabled, stroke related disability is common and its prevalence has been estimated at over 6/1,000 in the general population. In addition to its impact on the health of the population, stroke also imposes a huge cost on health services. Almost 5% of all health services costs in the UK and over 3% of the Dutch health care budget is attributed to stroke care. The lifetime costs of stroke were calculated 104,000 US Dollar for USA, 73,000 for Sweden and 60,000 US Dollar for Finland. However in Finland only 22,7% of the total lifetime costs were attributed to the acute care period of a stroke victim.

Stroke is a condition with high incidence and mortality rates, leaving a large proportion of survivors with significant residual physical, cognitive and psychological impairments. The increasing number of older adults and the emergence of new therapies for acute stroke suggest there will be an increase in the number of stroke survivors living with disabilities.

Most stroke patients show considerable recovery of function over the first few months. Although the exact extent and duration of this recovery is a matter of debate. Recovery occurs fastest in the first two weeks, by which time at least 50% of recovery has occurred but it is still continuing at following months (Wade et al., 1985).

All forms of rehabilitation aim to protect or restore personal and social identity. In this broad sense rehabilitation extends far beyond the bounds of medicine and within medicine all treatment processes are in some senses processes of rehabilitation.

Stroke rehabilitation is an active process beginning during acute hospitalisation, progressing for those with residual impairments to a systematic program of rehabilitation services and continuing after the individual returns to the community.

It is an organised effort to help stroke patients maximise all opportunities for returning to an active and productive lifestyle. Because the clinical manifestations of stroke are multifaceted and complex, stroke rehabilitation is best implemented through the co-ordinated efforts of a team of rehabilitation professionals (Gresham et al., 1997).

The rehabilitation process involves six major areas of focus:

(1) preventing, recognising and managing co-morbid illness and medical complications.
(2) training for maximum independence.
(3) facilitating, maximum, psychosocial coping and adaptation by patient and family.
(4) preventing secondary disability by promoting community reintegration, including resumption of home, family, recreational and vocational activities.
(5) enhancing quality of live in view of residual disability.
(6) preventing recurrent stroke and other vascular conditions such as myocardial infarction that occur with increased frequency in patients with stroke.

A rehabilitation management plan is the basis for all rehabilitation.

The first step is to match the patient with the appropriate rehabilitation services and setting. The primary criteria for rehabilitation are a reasonable medical stability, a significant functional disability and the ability to learn. Patients with severe cognitive deficits resulting in the inability to learn new strategies are unlikely to benefit from rehabilitation.

Several measures are used to assess, construct and evaluate the rehabilitation process over the recovery phases. During the acute phase of stroke baseline assessment should include standardised level of consciousness, a neurological deficit scale and a measure of global disability. In addition the type and severity of stroke, presence of co-morbidity and functional health patterns should be documented.

For documentation of severity of physical disability the best validated assessment instruments are the Barthel-index and the functional independence measure (FIM). These scales measure a range of activities essential to independence, including morbidity, self care and continence. For monitoring the rehabilitation process stroke deficit scales, cognitive screening tests, disability scales for ADL, motor, balance, morbidity, affect, language, speech, dysphagia, functionally oriented tests for cognition, functional health patterns and continence are used.

Measures of family functioning, instrumental activities of daily living (I-ADL's) and quality of live are helpful in documenting areas related to normal life patterns for those who return to the community. Instruments of stroke assessment are listed in Table 1 (Lyden and Lau, 1991).

General approach: stroke service and stroke units

There is now evidence that any nihilism which still surrounds stroke care is unjustified and that better organisation of inpatient stroke care improves patient outcomes and is probably cost effective (Jorgensen et al., 1999).

The term "stroke service" is a broad one and should incorporate the range of facilities required to provide comprehensive care of stroke. Functions of a comprehensive stroke service are:

Table 1. Measures for the rehabilitation process after stroke

Acute phase and screening for rehabilitation
Glasgow-Coma Scale and Mini-Mental-Status
NIH-Stroke Scale (Stroke Scale)
Rankin Scale (Disability Scale)
Barthel Index, FIM (ADL-Scale)
Chronic phase and monitoring rehabilitation
NIH-Stroke Scale
Cognitive screening
ADL Scale
Quality Life Scale

(1) stroke as an emergency
(2) organised prehospital management and immediate admission
(3) prompt and accurate diagnosis
(4) detailed assessment (cause of stroke, co-existing conditions, impairment, disability, handicap, social background)
(5) effective and appropriate medical or surgical treatment
(6) prevention and treatment of complications
(7) provision of neurorehabilitation
(8) secondary prevention and follow-up
(9) resettlement of patients at home or arrangements for institutional care
(10) education of staff
(11) quality assessment
(12) research

The crucial first step in setting a stroke service is to identify an individual who will take responsibility. There should be a widely circulated policy for a health care district. The service has to integrate hospital and community resources.

Several models for stroke services have been described. Stroke units have received special attention but are far from homogenous in different countries. It is clear that stroke units form only one part of a comprehensive stroke service although this is likely to be most important part (Sulch et al., 2000).

The type of stroke services that hospitals provide varies considerably from place to place.

The results of the systematic review provide good evidence that hospital based stroke services should be organised (Stroke Unit Trialist's Collaboration, 1997, 2000; Langhorne and Dennis, 1998; Langhorne and Duncan, 2001).

Patients managed in stroke units where more likely to survive, regain independence and return at home. The results of individual trials suggest that the stroke units may also improve the patients quality of live and that improvements in outcome persist for several years.

Descriptive studies have identified several distinctive features of stroke unit care which appear to have improved patient outcomes. These include the following: a co-ordinated multidisciplinary team care provided by a team of medical, nursing, physiotherapy, occupational therapy and social worker staff and co-ordinated through regular meetings — routine nursing care was closely linked with this multidisciplinary care; and a staff with a special interest in stroke or rehabilitation care and programmes of ongoing education and training in stroke (Ronning and Guldvog, 1998; Indredavik et al., 1998, 1999a,b).

About 50% of the trials in the meta-analysis were of acute stroke units whilst the rest where primarily of stroke rehabilitation units. Admitting all acute stroke patients directly into a unit makes the introduction of assessment protocols easier, allows expertise to be focused and will urgently facilitate the very large randomised trials of acute treatments that are needed to identify effective treatments.

Also admission of patients directly to an acute stroke unit facilitates a policy of aggressive early mobilisation, hydration, control of temperature, avoidance of hypoxia and large changes in blood pressure. Although there are no reliable data from randomised trials demonstrating that anyone of these interventions improves outcomes, they are supported by a reasonable theoretical rationale and some observational data.

Perhaps the most successful approach is the comprehensive stroke unit which admit patients acutely and then provide at least a few weeks of rehabilitation.

Such a model which is wide spread in Scandinavia is supported by several trials included in the systematic review.

It is of interest to look at the absolute outcome rates. Results can be calculated in terms of the number of adverse outcomes avoided by managing 100 patients in an organised stroke unit care setting. It is apparent that for every 100 patients managed in a stroke unit five more returned home in an independence state, four fewer died and one less was in institutional care (Table 2). Therefore stroke unit care was associated with an absolute increase in good outcomes without any substantial increase in the number of dependent survivors living either at home or in an institution.

Results can be calculated as the numbers who need to be managed in an organised stroke unit to prevent one adverse outcome, the number needed to treat — NNT. Using the data in Table 2 we can calculate that approximately 25 patients need to be treated to prevent one death while the NNT to ensure one extra patient returns home independent is 20. These results compare

Table 2. Absolute outcomes in the stroke unit trials

Outcome	SU	Control	OR (95% Ci)	Abs. Diff. 95% Ci
Death	23%	28%	0.8 (0.7–1.0)	−4 (−7–0)
Institutional Care	20%	22%	0.8 (0.7–1.0)	−1 (−4–+1)
Home (Dependent)	18%	16%	1.0 (0.7–1.4)	0 (−4–+3)
Home (Independent)	39%	33%	1.4 (1.2–1.7)	+5 (+1–+8)

favourable with many medical interventions. This information can also be used to carry out an economic analysis of stroke unit care.

No study has shown to what extension the beneficial effect is due to specific rehabilitation strategies, to the daily time spent in physiotherapy, occupational therapy or is it a non-specific effect of a more stimulating environment with competent staff that can encourage and support the patients and family members. Scientific evidence demonstrating the various specific rehabilitation interventions after stroke is limited. Comparisons between different methods in current use have so far failed to show that any particular stroke rehabilitation strategy is superior to another.

Specific approach

Facilitation of brain repair mechanisms

The surviving brain itself is responsible for the considerable functional recovery and reorganisation of the cortical network which is seen in patients after stroke when many genes regulating the trophic effects that govern neuronal growth, sprouting and synapse formation are induced.

Studies using PET, functional MRI, transcranial stimulation and magnetencephalography support a concept of functional reorganisation after stroke. PET-studies on blood flow distribution during finger movements in a previously paretic hand have demonstrated complex patterns of activation which increased activity with large individual variations (Weiller et al., 1992, 1993; Heiss et al., 1999; Kopp et al., 1999; Musso et al., 1999). Until now studies comparing the degree and pattern of activation in patients with good and less than good recovery and specific therapeutic interventions are few and the published data are sometimes contradictory. Because of large individual variations, careful longitudinal studies of individual patients with specific deficits and well-defined lesions are needed.

Independent of the infarct size, restorative therapies could significantly enhance the recovery by promoting functional compensation by surviving brain areas, stimulated neuronal sprouting or novel synaptic connections and other strategies affecting brain plasticity: an enriched environment that allowed the performance of various tasks after a brain insult was shown to facilitate recovery when rats where placed in the enriched environment immediately after the ischemic infarct and even when the transfer was delayed for two weeks, suggesting that a rich environment may stimulate mechanisms that enhance brain plasticity. Similar approaches have already been incorporated into rehabilitative approaches and are used in stroke units too.

Paradoxically, surviving tissue in the injured hemisphere may be fatally vulnerable to excessive behavioural demand. If the impaired limb is overused while the intact limb is restricted by a cast, injury size is greatly increased and recovery of function is severely disrupted. The use-it-or-lose-it rehabilitative approach is popular, but an over aggressive strategy should be avoided. However, it has been reported that changes in activation pattern can be induced by forced training of the paretic hand even for to fifteen years after stroke onset.

Which processes bring about spontaneous neurological recovery and can be enhanced by arm and leg rehabilitation?

Possible mechanisms include recovery of penumbral tissue around the infarcted area, subcortical reorganisation, reduction of temporally deactivated intact brain regains remote from but anatomically connected to the area of primary injury, including reinforcement of ipsilateral motor pathways such as thalamus, caudate, lentiform nuclei, prefrontal cortex; and behavioural compensations (Johansson, 2000).

Greater intensity of leg rehabilitation improves functional recovery and health-related functional status, whereas greater intensity of arm rehabilitation results in small improvements in dexterity, providing further evidence that exercise therapy primarily induces treatment effects on the abilities at which training is specifically aimed. In a randomised study of 101 patients Kwakkel et al. found that an additional 30 min. of therapy daily for 5 days a week for up to 20 weeks can make a substantial difference to functional recovery and that the effect is specific to the focus of the therapy. This benefit was achieved in the context of a total of one hour and 20 minutes of rehabilitation therapy daily. This study shows how great an effect a small quantity of a specific input may achieve (Kwakkel et al., 1999a,b; Dickstein, 1986). Physiotherapy is the main therapeutic option in hemiparesis although techniques vary (Ernst, 1990). The two broad approaches most commonly employed the facilitation and inhibition technique and the functional approach. There has been very little formal evaluation of the physiotherapy techniques. No definite conclusions about the relative merits of different approaches can be drawn. So some important questions about physiotherapy after stroke remain: when should physiotherapy start and how long should it continue? what is the optimum intensity of physiotherapy? which specific therapeutic interventions are the most effective? which patients gain most from physiotherapy and can we prospectively identify them? (Langhorne et al., 1996; Lincoln et al., 1984, 1999; Ottenbacher and Janell, 1993; Pollock et al., 2000).

Interventions aimed at reducing physical, cognitive and emotional impairments may all improve activities of daily living (ADL) function. However, there is increasing evidence from randomised controlled trials that occupational therapy including training and practice, the introduction of aids and appliances and alterations to the patients environment can also reduce dependency in ADL and handicap (Gilbertson et al., 2000; Gladman et al., 1995; Walker et al., 1999).

A large number of physical techniques have been developed with the aim of improving motor function or gait (Dean and Sheperd, 1997; Feys et al., 1998; Kwakkel et al., 1997; Kunkel et al., 1999; van der Lee, 1999). There are some small RCT's which have included highly selected patients and focused more on impairment than disability as outcome measures. Non are supported by enough evidence to recommend their routine news. Different types of biofeedback (EMG, visual and auditory feedback) may help patients achieve better sitting or standing balance (Burridge et al., 1997; Chae et al., 1998;

Glanz et al., 1995, 1996; Moreland et al., 1994, 1998; Schleenbacker et al., 1993).

Johansson et al. (2001) performed a multicenter randomised controlled trial where 115 patients with moderate or severe functional impairment where included. Patients were randomised to a acupuncture group, sensory stimulation with high intensity, low frequency transcutaneous electrical nerve stimulation group and to a control group receiving low intensity (subliminal high frequency electrical stimulation). When compared with a control group that received subliminal electrical stimulation, treatment during the subacute phase of stroke with acupuncture or transcutaneous electrical nerve stimulation with muscle contractions had no beneficial effects on functional outcome or live satisfaction (Johansson et al., 2001). Our research with functional magnetic resonance imaging has demonstrated that whole-hand stimulation at the subthreshold level for sensation may to some extent affect regional blood flow in the primary and secondary motor and somatosensory areas of the brain (Golazewski et al., 1998). Therefore in designing future trials of acupuncture after stroke having another control group with no intervention except conventional rehabilitation could provide supplementary information.

Current data on plasticity indicates that various types of training sensory stimulation and activation can influence rehabilitation. Functional electrical stimulation can reduce foot drop to facilitate gait, it probably increases muscle strength but it is unclear whether it improves functional outcome and many patients find it uncomfortable (Gosman-Hedstrom et al., 1998; Leandri et al., 1990; Price and Pandyan, 2000; Tekeoolu et al., 1998).

Estimates of the frequency of aphasia have inevitably depended on the population and screening methods used (Pederson et al., 1995). In the Oxfordshire community stroke project 19% of 564 assessable patients were found to be dysphasic at first assessment. Whilst in the hospital-based Copenhagen stroke study 38% of 881 conscious patients where judged dysphasic according to the Scandinavian stroke scale.

There is considerable controversy about the effectiveness of speech and language therapy in aphasia (Sellars et al., 2000). The results of the randomised control trials have been disappointing, mainly because of methodological weaknesses. Criticism include the failure to describe the interventions, use of weak or low intensity interventions, inappropriate control therapies, unblinded assessments of outcome and small numbers of patients, lost to follow-up or not complying with the treatment (Ferro et al., 1999).

Although some studies have shown that intensive treatment may be effective, others have shown now clear evidence of benefit from less intensive treatment.

Several small randomised control trials have shown that at least for selected patients similar outcomes can be achieved from the input of volonteers, working with guidance from a speech and language therapist vs. regular therapy from trained therapist. One meta-analysis of both randomised and non-randomised studies of the effectiveness of therapy on language concluded that therapy whether introduced early or late definitely enhanced spontaneous recovery. This meta-analysis also concluded that greater intensity of treatment produced larger effects (Roby, 1998).

Another systematic review but one which included only randomised trials was far more cautious in conclusion suggesting there was insufficient evidence of benefit (Greener et al., 1998, 2000a). Both reviewers agree however that more methodologically robust randomised controlled trials are required to identify specific interventions which are effective in increasing the rate of recovery of aphasia and in decreasing the residual impairment, disability and handicap.

Pharmacological interventions

Considering the many complex events that occur in post ischaemic brain, it is likely that the efficacy of a drug can vary with the post-ischaemic time, size and type of lesion and interactions with other therapeutic interventions.

The use of pharmacotherapy as an adjunct to physical therapy and speech therapy is not new (Feeney, 1998). If combined with test-specific-training, norepinephrine, amphetamine and other alpha-adrenergic stimulating drugs can enhance motor performance after unilateral ablation of sensory motor cortex and have also been shown to enhance the immunoreactivity to synaptic proteins after focal brain ischaemia (Goldstein, 1998).

There are few very small randomised controlled trials investigating the combination therapy of amphetamine and physiotherapy with contradictory results (Crisostomo et al., 1988; Sonde et al., 2001; Walker-Batson et al., 1995). In order to find a possible and optimal regime of amphetamine to enhance motor recovery without adverse effects, future clinical studies should use a higher and/or more frequent dosage of amphetamine as well as a longer treatment period together with a greater number of patients.

In addition to the effect of noradrenergic agents on motor recovery, several other classes of drugs that act on the CNS may affect recovery from other types of behavioural deficits. GABA agonists may have either negative or positive effects.

Depression is common after stroke and often prompts the use of antidepressant medications. The administration of a single dose of trazodone transiently slows motor recovery in rats with sensorimotor cortex injury and reinstates the hemiparesis in recovered animals. A single dose of desipramine facilitates motor recovery, in contrast fluoxetine and amitriptyllin have no demonstrable effect on motor recovery after experimental focal brain injury.

Dopaminergic agents may influence recovery from neglect caused by praefrontal cortical injury. Apomorphine, a dopamine agonist, reduces the severity of experimentally induced neglect. Concurrent administration of haloperidol also blocks amphetamine-promoted recovery and transiently reinstates the deficits in recovered animals.

The recent review and analysis by the Cochrane group of the controlled studies on the efficacy of speech therapy summarised this outcome literature

Table 3. Selected laboratory and clinical findings of drug effects on recovery after stroke

Drug	Effect	Laboratory recovery effect	Clinical recovery effect
Norepinephrine Bitartrate			
Amphetamine Sulfate	sympathomimetic	+	+
Phenylpropranolamine	sympathomimetic	+	No Data
Methylphenidate	sympathomimetic	+	?
Yohimbine	α_2 AR Antagonist	+	No Data
Clonidine	α_2 AR Antagonist	–	–
GABA			
Diazepam	Gabaagonist	–	–
Piracetam		–	+
Antidepressants			
Fluoxetine	5-HT Reuptake Blocker	+	No Data
Desipramine	NE Reuptake Blocker	+	No Data
Amitriptyline	Mixed 5 HT and NE Reuptake Neutral Blocker		No Data
Dopamine			
Haloperidol	Butyrophenone	–	–
Apomorphine	Agonist	+	No Data

as not been shown either to be clearly effective or clearly ineffective (Sellar et al., 2000). There is some evidence that drugs might improve language function or enhance the effects of language therapy (Greener et al., 2002b).

The Dallas group recently published a prospective double-blind study in which 21 affected patients where randomly asigned to receive either 10 mg dextro-amphetamine or placebo. One week after drug sections ended there was a significant difference in recovery between the groups. The results are unique compared to those typically conducted on the efficacy of rehabilitation treatments a decade earlier (Walker-Batson et al., 2001).

The most intensively studied drug is piracetam. The Cologne group recently published a prospective double-blind placebo controlled study investigating whether piracetam improves language recovery in post stroke aphasia assisted by neuropsychological tests and activation PET measurement of cerebral blood flow.

Before treatment, both groups were comparable with respect to performance in language tasks and to type and severity of aphasia. In the piracetam group, increase of activation effect was significantly higher in the left transverse temporal gyrus, left triangular part of inferior frontal gyrus and left posterior superior temporal gyrus after the treatment period compared with the initial measures. In the test battery the pirazetam group improved in six language functions, the placebo group only in three subtests. This study included calculation of more than 17 significance tests of the aphasia and neuropsychological tests and they do not report any alpha level adjustment

(Kessler et al., 2000). It is believed that there is currently to little evidence to recommend the use of pirazetam or other drugs outside randomised controlled trials.

Experimental approaches

Neural transplantation and neurogenesis: The studies using neural transplants to alleviate the effects of ischemic brain injury where initiated in the 1980's and 1990's. In MCA occlusion models in rats, fetal grafts were shown to survive and receive extensive innervation from the host, although the functional effects of the grafts in alleviating cognitive and sensorimotor deficits remain uncertain. Neuronal stem cells have been shown to improve stroke recovery in rats.

Implantation of fetal neocortical cells after cortical lesions have been performed successfully in several laboratories. Transplanted cells can interact with the host tissue by forming connections but also by being a source of trophic factors that can influence the surrounding tissue. Although both anatomic and functional integration with the host brain have been observed, improvement in behavioural tests have been noticed only when transplantation is combined with post transplantation housing in an enriched environment. If performed one week after ligation of MCA but not if delayed for three weeks, the combined procedure can improve functional outcome more than an enriched environment alone and it can also reduce the secondary thalamic atrophy that occurs after cortical lesions.

Although grafting can successfully be performed at later post ischaemic times, there is so far no evidence for functional improvement at later times (Mattson et al., 1997).

Neural stem cells, multipotential cells that are praecursors to neurons and glia, have been identified in the adult vertebrate central nervous system. Stem cells are also present in human brains shown in tissue cultures from the subependymal zone and periventricular white matter. Recent studies have shown, that they can differentiate to neurons in the adult human dentate gyrus in vivo. Stem cells from the adult brain proliferate and differentiate into neurons and glia in tissue culture with the same efficiency for neuronal differentiation as found in fetal stem cells (Eriksson et al., 1998). With the observation that such cells in experimental studies can be manipulated in vivo by growth factors and by environmental enrichment, the clinical potential of in vivo manipulation of stem cells in humans is currently subject to much speculation.

Endogenous growth factors may provide neuroprotection acutely and enhance neuronal sprouting later. Basic fibroblast growth factor reduces infarct size acutely and improves functional outcome in chronically treated rats. Phase II trials in the acute phase of stroke are ongoing, however, these trials were not designed to investigate whether the putative delayed therapeutic window, aiming at enhancement of the spontaneous restorative brain processes, can be used clinically. Other growth factors have shown neuroprotective effects in in vitro and in vivo experiments, and clinical studies with novel approaches will probably follow (Johansson, 1998).

Both basic and clinical research are critical to improving rehabilitation for stroke survivors. An increasing body of scientific evidence suggests that cortical function reorganisation occurs after central nervous system damage and that this reorganisation interacts with environmental influences that may facilitate functional recovery. Because rehabilitation seeks to enhance recovery after stroke, rehabilitation specialists are interested in investigating the neurological mechanisms of recovery and the mechanisms of skill reaquisition after stroke.

Major gaps in knowledge concerning the effectiveness of specific interventions to remedy at communication disorders, sensorimotor and cognitive perceptual impairments as well as those to restore functional independence remain. Relations between the site and extent of lesion, associated impairments, and the functional consequences need study to be adequately understood. Research is needed to establish the effects of a wide variety of rehabilitation therapies and interventions. Development of valid, standardised, reliable and sensitive measures of rehabilitation are the basis for such endeavours.

References

Burridge JH, Taylor PN, Hagan SA, Wood DE, Swain ID (1997) The effects of common peroneal stimulation on the effort and speed of walking: a randomised controlled trial with chronic hemiplegic patients. Clin Rehabil 11: 201–210

Chae J, Bethoux F, Bohine T, Dobos L, Davis T, Friedl, A (1998) Neuromuscular stimulation for upper extremity motor and functional recovery in acute hemiplegia. Stroke 29: 975–979

Crisostomo EA, Duncan PW, Propst M, Dawson DV, Davis JN (1988) Evidence that amphetamine with physical therapy promotes recovery of motor function in stroke patients. Ann Neurol 23: 94–97

Dean CM, Shepherd RB (1997) Task related training improves performance in seated reaching tasks after stroke. A randomised controlled trial. Stroke 28: 722–728

Dickstein R, Hocherman S, Pillar T, Shaham, R (1986) Stroke rehabilitation. Three exercise therapy approaches. Phys Ther 66: 1233–1238

Eriksson PS, Perfilieva E, Björk-Eriksson T, Alborn, A-M, Nordborg C, Peterson DA, Gage FH (1998) Neurogenesis in the adult human hippocampus. Nat Med 4: 1313–1317

Ernst E (1990) A review of stroke rehabilitation and physiotherapy. Stroke 21: 1081–1085

Feeney DM (1998) Mechanisms of noradrenergic modulation of physical therapy: effects on functional recovery after cortical injury. In: Goldstein LB (ed) Restorative neurology: advances in pharmacotherapy for recovery after stroke. Futura Publishing Co, Armonk, pp 35–78

Ferro JM, Mariano G, Madureira S (1999) Recovery from aphasia and neglect. Cerebrovasc Dis 9 [Suppl 5]: 6–22

Feys HM, De Weerdt WJ, Selz BE et al (1998) Effect of a therapeutic intervention for the hemiplegic upper limb in the acute phase after stroke. A single blind, randomised, controlled multicentre trial. Stroke 29: 785–792

Gilbertson L, Langhorne P, Walker A, Allen, A (2000) Domiciliary occupational therapy for stroke patients discharged home from hospital: a randomised controlled trial. Br Med J 320: 603–606

Gladman JRF, Lincoln NB, Barer DH (1993) A randomised controlled trial of domiciliary and hospital-based rehabilitation for stroke patients after discharge from hospital. J Neurol Neurosurg Psychiatry 56: 960–966

Glanz M, Klawansky S, Stason W et al (1995) Biofeedback therapy in post-stroke rehabilitation: a meta-analysis of the randomised controlled trials. Arch Phys Med Rehabil 76: 508–515

Glanz M, Klawansky S, Stason W, Berkey C, Chalmers TC (1996) Functional electrical stimulation in post-stroke rehabilitation: a meta-analysis of the randomised controlled trials. Arch Phys Med Rehabil 77: 549–553

Golaszewski S, Kremser C, Wagner M, Felber S, Aichner F, Dimitrijevic MM (1999) Functional magnetic resonance imaging of the human motor cortex before and after whole-hand afferent electrical stimulation. Scand J Rehabil Med 31: 165–173

Goldstein LB (1998) Potential effects of common drugs on stroke recovery. Arch Neurol 55: 454–456

Gosman-Hedstrom G, Claesson L, Klingenstierna U et al (1998) Effects of acupuncture treatment on daily life activities and quality of life. A controlled prospective, and randomised study of acute stroke patients. Stroke 29: 2100–2108

Greener J, Enderby P, Whurr R, Grant A (1998) Treatment for aphasia following stroke; evidence for effectiveness. Int J Language Commun Disord 33: 158–161

Greener J, Enderby P, Whurr R (2000a) Speech and language therapy for aphasia following stroke (Protocol for a Cochrane Review). In: The Cochrane Library. Updage Software, Oxford

Greener J, Enderby P, Whurr R (2000b) Pharmacological treatment for aphasia following stroke (Protocol for a Cochrane Review). In: The Cochrane Library. Update Software, Oxford

Gresham GE, Alexander D, Bishop DS, Giuliani C, Goldberg G, Holland A, Kelly-Hayes M, Linn RT, Roth EJ, Stason WB, Trombly CA (1997) Rehabilitation. Stroke 28: 1522–1526

Heiss WD, Kessler J, Thiel A, Ghaemi M, Karbe H (1999) Differential capacity of left and right hemispheric areas for compensation of poststroke aphasia. Ann Neurol 45: 430–438

Indredavik B, Bakke F, Slordahl SA, Rokseth R, Haheim LL (1998) Stroke unit treatment improves long-term quality of life: a randomised controlled trial. Stroke 29: 895–899

Indredavik B, Bakke F, Slordahl SA, Rokseth R, Haheim LL (1999a) Stroke unit treatment: 10 year follow up. Stroke 30: 1524–1527

Indredavik B, Bakke F, Slordahl SA, Rokseth R, Haheim LL (1999b) Treatment in a combined acute and rehabilitation stroke unit: which aspects are most important? Stroke 30: 917–923

Johansson BB (1998) Neurotrophic factors and transplants. In: Goldstein LB (ed) Restorative neurology: advances in pharmacotherapy for recovery after stroke. Futura Publishing Co, Armonk, pp 141–166

Johansson BB (2000) Brain plasticity and stroke rehabilitation. Stroke 31: 223–230

Johansson BB, Haker E, von Arbin M, Britton M, Langström G, Terént A, Ursing D, Asplund K (2001) Acupuncture and transcutaneous nerve stimulation in stroke rehabilitation, a randomised controlled trial. Stroke 32: 707–713

Jorgensen HS, Kammersgaard LP, Nakayama H, et al (1999) Treatment and rehabilitation on a stroke unit improves 5-year survival: a community-based study. Stroke 30: 930–933

Kessler J, Thiel A, Karbe H, Heiss WD (2000) Piracetam improves activated blood flow and facilitates rehabilitation of poststroke aphasic patients. Stroke 31: 2112–2116

Kopp B, Kunkel A, Muhlnickel W, Villringer K, Taub E, Flow H (1999) Plasticity in the motor system related to therapy-induced improvement of movement after stroke. Neuroreport 10: 807–810
Kunkel A, Kopp B, Muller G, Villringer K, Villringer A, Taub E, Flor H (1999) Constraint-induced movement therapy for motor recovery in chronic stroke patients. Arch Phys Med Rehabil 80: 624–628
Kwakkel G, Wagenaar RC, Koelman TW, Lankhorst GJ, Koetsier JC (1997) Effects of intensity of rehabilitation after stroke. A research synthesis. Stroke 28: 1550–1556
Kwakkel G, Kollen BJ, Wagenaar RC (1999a) Therapy impact on functional recovery in stroke rehabilitation. Physiotherapy 85: 377–391
Kwakkel G, Wagenaar RC, Twisk JWR, Lankhorst GJ, Koetsier JC (1999b) Intensity of leg and arm training after primary middle-cerebral-artery stroke: a randomised trial. Lancet 354: 191–196
Langhorne P, Dennis M (1998) Stroke units: an evidence based approach. BMJ Books, London
Langhorne P, Duncan P (2001) Does the organisation of postacute stroke care really matter? Stroke 32: 268–274
Langhorne P, Wagenaar R, Partridge C (1996) Physiotherapy after stroke: more is better? Physiother Res Int 1: 75–88
Leandri M, Parodi CI, Corrieri H, Rigardo S (1990) Comparison of TENS treatments in hemiplegic shoulder pain. Scand J Rehabil Med 22: 69–71
van der Lee JH, Wagenaar RC, Lankhorst GJ, Vogelaar TW, Deville WL, Bouter LM (1999) Forced use of the upper extremity in chronic stroke patients: results from a single-blind randomised clinical trial. Stroke 30: 2369–2375
Lincoln NB, Mulley GP, Jones AC, McGuirk E, Lendrem W, Mitchell RA (1984) Effectiveness of speech therapy for aphasic stroke patients. A randomised controlled trial. Lancet i: 1197–1200
Lincoln NB, Parry RH, Vass CD (1999) Randomised, controlled trial to evaluate increased intensity of physiotherapy treatment of arm function after stroke. Stroke 30: 573–579
Lyden PD, Lau GT (1991) A critical appraisal for stroke evaluation and rating scales. Stroke 22: 1345–1352
Mattsson B, Srensen HC, Zimmer J, Johansson BB (1997) Neural grafting to experimental neocortical infarcts improves behavioral outcome and reduces thalamic atrophy in rats housed in enriched but not in standard environments. Stroke 28: 1225–1232
Moreland JD, Thomson MA (1994) Efficacy of electromyographic biofeedback compared with conventional physical therapy for upper-extremity function in patients following stroke: a research overview and meta-analysis. Phys Ther 74: 534–547
Moreland JD, Thomson MA, Fuoco AR (1998) Electromyographic biofeedback to improve lower extremity function after stroke: a meta-analysis. Arch Phys Med Rehabil 79: 134–140
Musso M, Weiller C, Kiebel S, Muller SP, Bulau P, Rinjtjes M (1999) Training-induced brain plasticity. Brain 122: 1781–1790
Ottenbacher KJ, Jannell S (1993) The results of clinical trials in stroke rehabilitation research. Arch Neurol 50: 37–44
Pedersen PM, Jorgensen HS, Nakayama H, Raaschou HO, Olsen TS (1995) Aphasia in acute stroke: incidence, determinants, and recovery. Ann Neurol 38: 659–666
Pollock A, Langhorne P, Baer G (2000) Physiotherapy for the recovery of postural control and lower limb function following stroke (Protocol for a Cochrane Review). In: The Cochrane Library. Update Software, Oxford
Powell J, Pandyan AD, Granat M, Cameron M, Stott DJ (1999) Electrical stimulation of wrist extensors in post-stroke hemiplegia. Stroke 30: 1384–1389
Price CIM, Pandyan AD (2000) Electrical stimulation for preventing and treating post-stroke shoulder pain (Protocol for a Cochrane Review). In: The Cochrane Library. Update Software, Oxford

Roby RR (1998) A meta-analysis of clinical outcomes in the treatment of aphasia. J Speech Hearing Res 41: 172–187

Ronning OM, Guldvog B (1998) Outcome of subacute stroke rehabilitation: a randomised controlled trial. Stroke 29: 779–784

Schleenbaker RE, Mainous AGI (1993) Electromyographic biofeedback for the neuromuscular re-education in the hemiplegic stroke patient: a meta-analysis. Arch Phys Med Rehabil 74: 1301–1304

Sellars C, Hughes T, Langhorne P (2000) Speech and language therapy for dysarthria due to non-progressive brain damage. (Protocol for a Cochrane Review). In: The Cochrane Library. Update Software, Oxford

Sonde L, Nordström M, Nilsson CG, Lökk J, Viitanen M (2001) A double-blind placebo-controlled study of the effects of amphetamine and physiotherapy after stroke. Cerebrovasc Dis 12: 253–257

Stroke Unit Trialists'Collaboration (1997) Collaborative systematic review of the randomised trials of organised inpatient (stroke unit) care after stroke. Br Med J 314: 1151–1159

Stroke Unit Trialists'Collaboration (2000) Organised inpatient (stroke unit) care for stroke. In: The Cochrane Library. Update Software, Oxford

Sulch D, Peraz I, Melbourn A, Kalra L (2000) Randomised controlled trial of integrated (managed) care pathway for stroke rehabilitation. Stroke 31: 1929–1934

Tekeoolu Y, Adak B, Goksoy T (1998) Effect of transcutaneous electrical nerve stimulation (TENS) on Barthel Activities of Daily Living (ADL) index score following stroke. Clin Rehabil 12: 277–280

Wade DT, Wood VA, Langton Hewer R (1985) Recovery after stroke — the first 3 months. J Neurol Neurosurg Psychiatry 48: 7–13

Walker MF, Gladman JRF, Lincoln NB, Siemonsma P, Whitely T (1999) Occupational therapy for stroke patients not admitted to hospital: a randomised controlled trial. Lancet 354: 278–280

Walker-Batson D, Smith P, Curtis S, Unwin H, Greenlee R (1995) Amphetamine paired with physical therapy accelerates motor recovery after stroke. Further evidence. Stroke 26: 2254–2259

Walker-Batson D, Curtis S, Natarajan R, Ford J, Dronkers N, Salmeron E, Lai J, Unwin DH (2001) A double-blind, placebo-controlled study of the use of amphetamine in the treatment of aphasia. Stroke 32: 2093–2098

Weiller C, Chollet KJ, Friston KJ, Wise RJS, Frackowiak RSJ (1992) Functional reorganisation of the brain in recovery from striatocapsular infarction in man. Ann Neurol 31: 463–472

Weiller C, Ramsay SC, Wise RJS, Friston KJ, Frackowiak RSJ (1993) Individual patterns of functional reorganisation in the human cerebral cortex after capsular infarction. Ann Neurol 33: 181–189

Authors' address: Univ-Prof. Dr. F. Aichner, Department of Neurology, Wagner-Jauregg Hospital, Linz, Teaching Hospital, University Innsbruck, Wagner-Jauregg Weg 15, A-4021 Linz, Austria, e-mail: Franz.Aichner@wj.lkh.ooe.gv.at

J Neural Transm (2002) [Suppl] 63: 75–90

CADASIL and genetics of cerebral ischaemia

R. N. Kalaria, W. C. Low, A. E. Oakley, J. Y. Slade, P. G. Ince, C. M. Morris, and **T. Mizuno**

Institute for Ageing and Health, and Department of Psychiatry, University of Newcastle upon Tyne, United Kingdom

Summary. Recent advances suggest the existence of several autosomal dominantly inherited forms of cerebrovascular disorders. Mutations in diverse genes may induce direct pathological changes in intracranial vessels to cause cerebral ischaemic or haemorrhagic strokes leading to cognitive impairment and dementia. Similar pathology may also be caused by systemic vascular disease resulting from mutations and polymorphisms in genes that regulate cardiovascular physiology, blood coagulation and metabolic functions. The most common form of familial stroke appears to be CADASIL or cerebral autosomal dominant arteriopathy with subcortical infarcts and leukoencephalopathy. CADASIL is an arterial disease that has been linked to nucleotide substitutions and deletions in the *Notch* 3 gene. The pathogenesis of the disorder or how the mutations lead to cerebral infarcts and dementia is not known. However, elucidation of the microvascular pathology associated with such genetic disorders not associated with physiological risk factors for cardiovascular disease or stroke can bear much light on primary vascular mechanisms that lead to ischaemic blood flow and neuronal vulnerability.

Introduction

Cerebrovascular disease is a consequence of impairment of the blood supply to the brain. Ischaemic strokes account for 80% whereas intracerebral or subarachnoid haemorrhages constitute the rest of cerebrovascular disease (Kalimo et al., 1997). Cerebral infarction provoked by diminished oxygen and glucose availability may result from systemic vascular disease through large vessel emboli and atheromas or intracranial vascular disease. On the other hand hypertension is a frequent cause of cerebral haemorrhages. The extent of ischaemic damage will depend on the type, size and distribution of vessels as well as degree of insult. Oligaemia (hypoperfusion) occurring in the fringes of the ischaemic core (penumbra) or more widely upon impaired autoregulation of cerebral perfusion may lead to further irreversible injury if sustained over a long period.

The genetics of cerebrovascular disorders was virtually unknown until recently. They may have evaded genetic association because of widely variable phenotypes even within single gene disorders. A number of conditions within cerebrovascular disorders are recognized to be inherited in an autosomal dominant fashion. Hereditary forms of cerebrovascular disorders constitute only a small proportion (<10%) but they invariably cause extreme morbidity and mortality in both young and old. Causal genes and mutations linked to distinct cerebrovascular pathologies have been identified for several disorders directly affecting vessel structure and function (Kalaria, 2001). These have been variably termed vasculopathies and more precisely designated as angiopathies, arteriopathies and rarely endotheliopathies.

Inherited disorders that affect cardiac pathophysiology, thrombosis, haemostasis and mitochondrial functions are also of increased interest as causes of cerebrovascular disease. Pathogenic mutations and gene polymorphisms (allelic forms) in a wide variety of genes that play regulatory roles in systemic vascular and metabolic functions have been recognised (Hassan and Markus, 2000). These rather more complex group of single gene and polygenic diseases may be influenced by various factors including age, gender, race, and pre-existing vascular disease. However, focal neurological deficits and cognitive impairment could result irrespective of the etiology and pathogenesis. This short review considers cerebral autosomal dominant arteriopathy with subcortical infarcts and leukoencephalopathy (CADASIL) in the context of other angiopathies and arteriopathies. The elucidation of the genetics and pathogenesis of disorders such as CADASIL are important in understanding the primary vascular mechanisms that lead to ischaemic blood flow and its consequences on neuronal vulnerability.

CADASIL: a common form of familial stroke

Several hereditary conditions presenting with ischaemic strokes or focal infarcts unrelated to the amyloid angiopathies have been apparent (Table 1). The molecular genetics of familial disorders including the leukoencehalopathies (Leys et al., 1999; Adair et al., 1998; Utatsu et al., 1997; Grand et al., 1988; Gutman et al., 1989; Weil et al., 1999), rare occlusive conditions such as hereditary endotheliopathy retinopathy nephropathy with stroke or HERNS (Jen et al., 1997) and Moya-Moya (Ikeda et al., 1999; Yamauchi et al., 2000; Inoue et al., 2000) remain to be elucidated. These would be important in understanding ischaemic white matter pathology associated with brain haemorrhages and post-stroke dementia syndromes (Leys et al., 1999).

CADASIL emerges as the most common hereditary form of stroke leading to progressive dementia (Chabriat et al., 1995; Dichgans et al., 1998; Kalaria et al., 2000). CADASIL like disorders were first described as hereditary multi-infarct dementia (Sourander and Walinder, 1977) or chronic familial vascular encephalopathy (Stevens et al., 1977). Although the latter proved to be *Notch* 3 type CADASIL the Swedish hereditary disorder despite much similarity (Zhang et al., 1994) does not appear to be associated with *Notch* 3 mutations (Kalaria et al., unpublished observations). In view of the striking

Table 1. Inheritance of cerebrovascular disease

Group	Specific types	Genetics (gene/Chr)
Stroke(s)	CADASIL, Non-Notch vasculopathis, HERNS	*Notch* 3 and other genes various Chrs
Hypertensive angiopathies	Familial Binswanger's/ Leukoencephalopathies	unknown
Amyloid angiopathies	Icelandic, Dutch, Flemish, Prion, Finnish, Hungarian, British, Danish, Others	*Cystain C, AβPP, PrP, Gelsolin, TTR, BRI APOE*
Other angiopathies	Moyamoya disease	Gene unknown/Chr 3
Aneurysms	Sacular (berry), large aneurysms	Genes unknown (also congenital forms)
Vascular malformations CCMs	Cavernous angiomas	*KRIT1* and other genes on Chr 7 and 3 Ioci

AβPP amyloid precursor protein; *APOE* apolipoproteinE; *BRI* British dementia protein; *CCM* cerebral cavernous malformations; *Chr* chromosome; *HERNS* hereditary endotheliopathy retinopathy nephropathy with stroke; *Prp* prion protein; *TTR* transthyretin

white matter pathology and recurrent infarction CADASIL has also been considered a familial form of Binswanger's disease albeit in the absence of hypertension or hypercholestremia.

Current searches reveal that CADASIL appears to be far more common than previously perceived. It may be often overlooked and possibly misdiagnosed because it can present under various guises. CADASIL and its immediate variants consistently presenting with recurrent strokes and progressive dementia likely exist in over 500 families worldwide (Caronti et al., 1998; Chabriat et al., 1995; Bergmann et al., 1996; De Lange et al., 1999; Desmond et al., 1998; Lammie et al., 1995; Thomas et al., 2000). CADASIL cases have been identified in most countries of Western Europe, the Americas, Japan, Australia, the Caribbean and North Africa. There appear to be several families in the Nordic countries and at least 50 in the United Kingdom and in France, where the first linkage analysis had revealed the involvement of a locus on chromosome 19 subsequently identified to be the *Notch* 3 gene (product Notch 3) (Joutel et al., 1996).

Clinical features and brain imaging of CADASIL

CADASIL exhibits considerable phenotypic variability with thus far no clear relation to genotype (Chabriat et al., 1995; Hedera and Friedland, 1997; Salloway et al., 1998; Desmond et al., 1999; Malandrini et al., 1997). The disorder is invariably characterised by a history of migrainous attacks, followed by a series of subcortical strokes, signs of mood disorder in form of depression and cognitive disabilities. Migraine in CADASIL can be confused with familial hemiplegic migraine (Tournier-Lasserve, 1999), a channelopathy involving a different gene locus close to *Notch* 3. The average age of onset for CADASIL is 45 years (Chabriat et al., 1995). The recurrent stroke-like episodes may increase up to eight in the second decade after onset. Motor deficits, an ataxic hemiparesis, hemianopsia and dysarthria may accompany these principal events. Other features may include seizures, incomplete cerebellar ataxia, pseudobulbar palsy and unexplained coma. Neocortical strokes may also occur in some patients but they usually do not cover a wide territory. Large artery infarcts such as those of the middle or posterior cerebral artery are uncommon. The described features collectively lead to a rapidly progressing dementia, which appears severely manifest in the older patients (Dichgans et al., 1998). Psychiatric symptoms including confused mental states, severe forms of depression and signs of frontal dysfunction are manifest in more than 30% of the patients. CADASIL could also masquerade as a bipolar disorder.

The cerebrospinal fluid (CSF) from CADASIL patients reveals oligoclonal bands but these seem indistinguishable from those in other disorders. However, there may be CSF proteins of much interest (Dichgans et al., 1999a). Unlu et al. (2000) reported increased presence of factor B of the alternative complement pathway but it is likely that other modifying factors either genetic or epigenetic contribute to the phenotypic variations in age at onset, number of cerebrovascular incidents, degree of dementia and general morbidity. While these variable features seem unlikely due to an incomplete penetrance of the defective gene, the presence of migraine with visual aura in CADASIL along with a history of recurrent strokes are critical for the differential diagnosis of the disorder and distinguish CADASIL from multiple sclerosis, atypical Alzheimer's disease and Binswanger's disease, which exhibit white matter abnormalities upon magnetic resonance imaging (MRI).

The MR images reveal profound hyperintensities as white matter lesions and periventricular abnormalities in the basal ganglia, thalamus and external capsules (Maladrini et al., 1997; Chabriat et al., 1998; Yousry et al., 1999; Dichgans et al., 1999b). Our recent studies in a large English family revealed profound hyperintensities in the deep white matter in affected patients compared to the unaffected (Coulthard et al., 2000). These lesions also observed in the corpus callosum appear secondary to small vessel disease. The hypersignals interpreted as ischaemic infarcts, lacunes and a diffuse leukoencephalopathy increase exponentially after the age of 40 (Filley et al., 1999). Ventricular dilatation similar to that seen in Alzheimer's and Binswanger's diseases is not usually evident in CADASIL. While the images are often mistaken for demeylinating disease, MRI is thought to provide almost 100% sensitivity especially if the clinical diagnostic criteria are satisfied. White matter lesions are most readily detected with FLAIR sequences and abnormalities in the temporal pole appear most characteristic (Fig. 1). There appear to be only a couple of positron emission tomography (PET) studies on CADASIL (Mellies et al., 1998). The PET studies essentially confirm the remarkable deficits in cerebral blood flow and glucose consumption in asymptomatic patients that are sustained during the subsequent phase but are accompanied by decreases in the oxygen extraction fraction. Future imaging studies should identify the structural substrates of the associated dementia

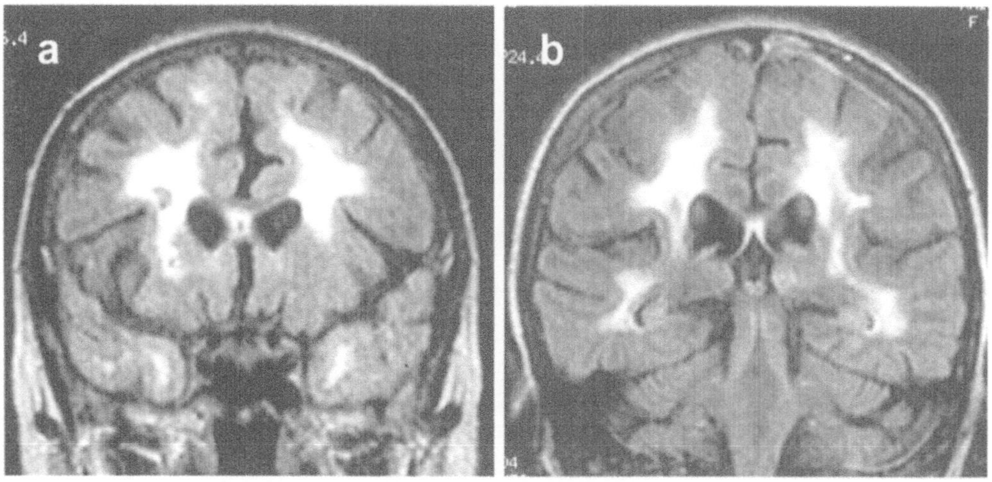

Fig. 1. FLAIR sequences on MRI in a CADASIL patient with a mutation in exon 4 of Notch 3. Note in **a** clear hyperintense signals in temporal poles in addition to involvement of the centrum semiovale region. Scans by courtesy of Dr Cleland, Sunderland Hospital

and provide proof for cerebral atrophy beyond the accepted notions that hyperintensities represent disconnection between the subcortical and cortical structures or disruption of cortico-cortical pathways. The few neuropsychological studies using a battery of modified tests as those applied in Alzheimer's disease suggest that CADASIL patients undergo a gradual cognitive decline accompanied by a motor slowness and rigidity as well loss of executional functions (Trojano et al., 1998; Tuominen et al., 2001).

In accord with currently recognized treatments for cerebrovascular disease, strategies that would enhance cerebral reperfusion are recommended for CADASIL. The use of anticoagulants and thrombolytic agents such as warfarin and heparin would not be considered appropriate in fear of bleeding. Despite perhaps low efficacy in some patients aspirin is the best choice as a prophylactic and has the advantage of being associated with the least number of complications. The long term use of neuroprotective agents such as N-methyl D-aspartate antagonists and agents that act via other mechanisms such as voltage sensitive calcium channel antagonists, for example nimopidine and flunarizine have also been suggested. Recent advances in the therapeutics of Alzheimer's disease suggest the use of novel compounds like propentofylline, a xanthine derivative with multiple actions, is beneficial even in vascular dementia. This might be an effective strategy for retaining good cerebral perfusion and enhancing energy stores in CADASIL sufferers.

Cerebrovascular pathology in CADASIL

CADASIL bears a distinct cerebrovascular pathology. In contrast to cerebral amyloid angiopahty (CAA) vascular abnormalities also occur in peripheral tissues (Ruchoux and Murage, 1997; Kalimo et al., 1999). Cerebral atrophy

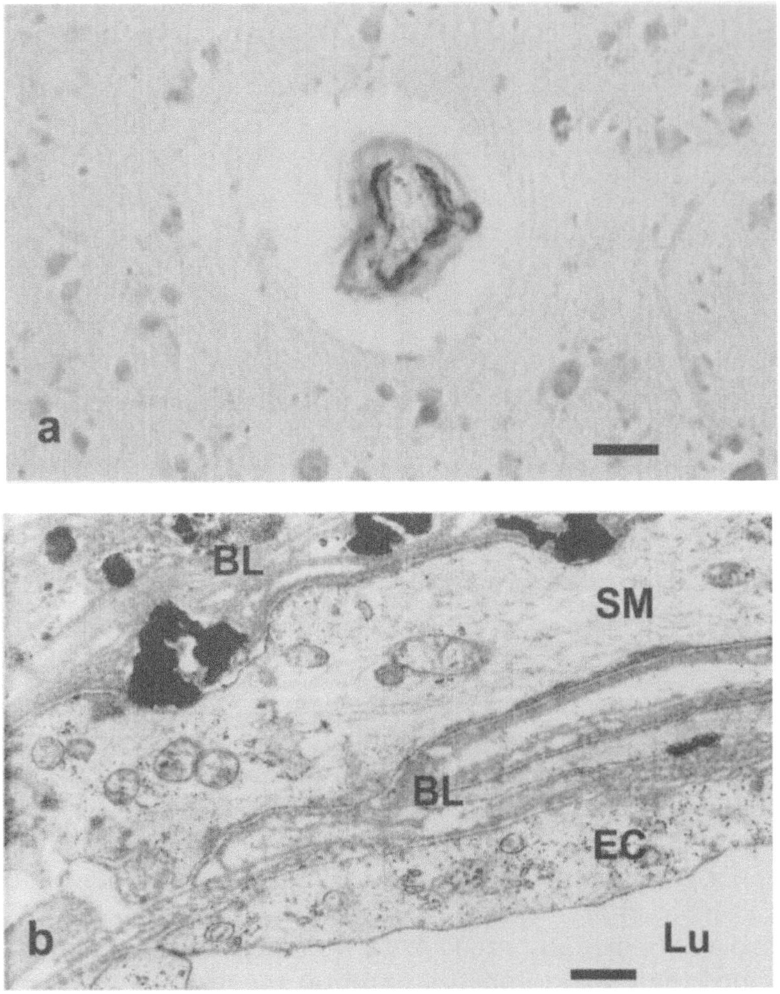

Fig. 2. Microvascular pathology in cerebral vessels from a CADASIL patient with confirmed Notch 3 mutation (R153C). **a** shows disruption of alpha-actin immunoreactive vascular smooth cells within the medial layers. Also note marked depletion of perivascular neuronal density. Counterstain with Nissl; **b** electron micrograph from a cerebral arteriole showing deposits (asterisks) of granular osmiophilic material (GOM). Recent studies have suggested that both programmed cell death and inflammatory markers such as caspase 3 like reactivity and complement 3 are also evident in the vessel wall afflicted in CADASIL (WC Low et al., unpublished observations). *BL* basal lamina; *EC* endothelial cell; *Lu* lumen; *SM* smooth muscle cell. Magnification bar **a** = 200 um; **b** = 500 nm

has been described in some cases but has not been widely confirmed. The lumen of cerebral microvessels is consistently narrowed through unrelenting intimal thickening and expansion of the extracellular matrix. This is accompanied by widespread disruption and degeneration of smooth muscle cells in vessel wall (Fig. 2). Despite severe vascular degeneration haemorrhages are not apparent. Perivascular fibrosis and intimal changes presumably fortify and reseal the vessel wall preventing disintegration. Both intracranial and extracranial arterial vessels may acquire 1–2 μm size extracellular granular osmiophilic deposits (Ruchoux and Murage, 1997), which remain to be characterised (Fig. 2b). They may be lipophilic but do not contain Notch 3 fragments (Joutel et al., 2000a). Recent immunochemical studies suggest that perhaps consistent with the shedding of the extracellular portion of the heterodimeric receptor (cf. Fig. 4) the walls of cerebral arteries, arterioles and capillaries in CADASIL accumulate the larger ~200 kD epidermal growth factor repeat (EGF) containing domain of Notch 3 (Joutel et al., 2000a).

Why may CADASIL be considered a CNS disorder if the vasculopathy is also consistently evident in peripheral tissues? Unlike the systemic vasculature, cerebral arterioles and capillaries are not fenestrated and endowed a "tight" cerebral endothelium. The muscular and endothelial abnormalities in cerebral vessels (Kalaria, 1996) of both the subcortical grey and white matter would be detrimental to the blood brain barrier properties (Ruchoux and Murage, 1997). Degeneration of penetrating arteries and arterioles would have severe repercussions on subcortical blood flow to the white matter with consequences on cerebral function.

Molecular genetics of Notch 3 and CADASIL

More than 80% of the first identified familial cases with atypical headache or stroke in young adults were thought to be sporadic (Chabriat et al., 1998). Although autosomal dominant inheritance of CADASIL may not be obvious single missense mutations in the *Notch* 3 gene (Joutel et al., 1996, 1997; Oberstein et al., 1999; Kamimira et al., 1999; Escary et al., 2000) co-segregate with disease. *Notch* 3 is one of at least four genes, which encode single-pass transmembrane (TM) cell surface receptors of ~300 kDa. The receptor protein embodies 2,321 amino acids integrated as 34 tandem epidermal growth factor-like (EGF) repeats, 3 cysteine rich Notch/lin-12 repeats and 6 cdc 10/ankhyrin repeats (Fig. 3). A PEST (for proline, glutamate, serine and threonine) is also present at the carboxyl terminal. Notch proteins that regulate cell fates or control the ability of non-terminally differentiated cells to respond to proliferation and maturation signals, through local cell interactions (Artavanis-Tsakonas et al., 1999; Weinmaster, 1997). Co-expression of Notch proteins and presenilins (PS) in adult CNS and vascular cells suggests an essential role for Notch in a different capacity such as programmed cell death. Studies in *caenorhabditis elegans* show that LIN-12, a Notch homologue interacts with SEL-12. PS 1 as the human homologue of SEL-12 can also suppress LIN-12 activity but the mutated PS1, implicated in familial AD is unable to achieve similar degree of effect (Kimble and Simpson, 1997; Shimizu et al., 1999).

The *Notch* 3 gene assumes 33 exons (Fig. 3, indicated by boxes). There appear more than 60 different mutations in *Notch* 3 (Table 2). Most of the mutations are clustered upstream (exon 4) within the extracellular EGF repeat region and singularly involve either loss or gain of cysteine residues (Joutel et al., 1997; Escary et al., 2000). However, small in-frame shift dele-

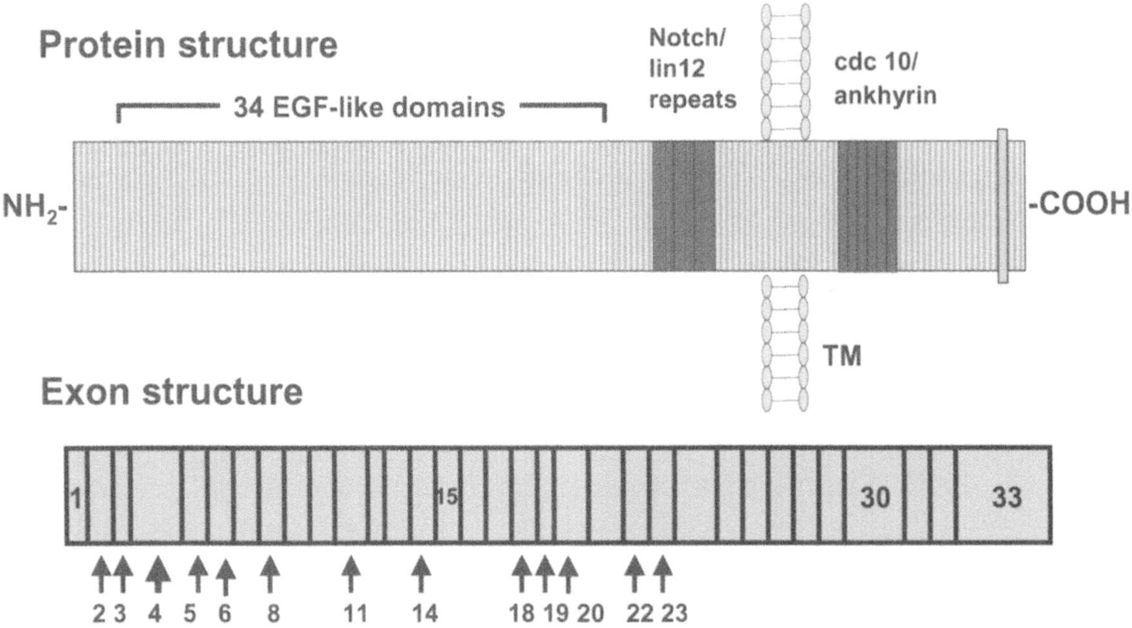

Fig. 3. Structures of the Notch 3 protein (above) and the gene (below) showing the extracellular and intracellular domains (modified from Joutel et al., 1997; Kalimo et al., 1999). Arrows indicate exons in which mutations have been found (see Table 2). A large cluster of the single missense mutations all involving an amino acid change from or to cysteine is localised to exons 4 and 5. Expression studies using primer sequences from exons 30–33 show that Notch 3 mRNA is readily expressed in cerebral vessels and vascular smooth muscle cells (Mizuno et al., unpublished results)

tions created by splice site mutations have also been reported that too alter the number of cysteine residues (Table 2b; Joutel et al., 2000b; Dichgans et al., 2000). A heterozygous *de novo* mutation (Arg to Cys in codon 182) has been described emphasizing that possible diagnosis of CADASIL may not be rejected in the absence of family history (Joutel et al., 2000c).

How does the defect in *Notch* 3 gene produce clinical symptoms and pathology of CADASIL? To consider this it is pertinent to understand the ligand-induced Notch signalling and cleavage of the receptor in vertebrates (Fig. 4). Interactions between Jagged 1 (a DSL for Delta/Serrate/LAG-2) ligand and Notch expressing cells lead to activation of Notch signalling in the receiving cells. Jagged 1 may bind multiple Notch receptors and interacts with the Notch EGF motif between exons 10 and 12. As a result of ligand binding, Notch intracellular domain (NICD) undergoes nuclear translocation and binds to RBP-jk transcription factor to activate or repress regulatory sequences of the (Hairy) enhancer of split (HES) complex genes. Post translation and proteolytic events may regulate activities of the Notch receptor prior to nuclear activation (Artvanis-Tsakonas et al., 1999). Notch undergoes cellular events that resemble those involved in cleavage of APP; receptor is apparently cleaved in the trans-Golgi network by a Furin-like convertase (Annaert and De Strooper, 1999) between the LIN-12 and transmembrane domains and

Table 2.a. Currently known mutations in Notch 3 linked to CADASIL

No	EGF Domain	Amino acid change	Exon	Notch 3 nucleotide change	% of mutations per exon*
1	1	Cys 49 Tyr	2	tGt 224 tAt	3.3
2		Arg 54 Cys		Cgt 238 Tgt	
3		Trp 71 Cys	3	tgG 291 tgT	8.3
4		Cys 76 Arg		Tgt 304 Cgt	
5	2	Arg 90 Cys		Cgt 346 Tgt	
6		Cys 93 Phe		tGc 356 tTc	
7		Arg 110 Cys		Cgt 406 Tgt	
8		Cys 117 Phe	4	tGc 428 tTc	53.0
9	3	Cys 123 Phe		tGc 446 tTc	
10		Cys 123 Tyr		tGc 446 tAc	
11		Arg 133 Cys		Cgc 475 Tgc	
12		Cys 134 Trp		tgC 480 tgG	
13		Arg 141 Cys		Cgc 499 Tgc	
14		Phe 142 Cys		tTc 503 tGc	
15		Cys 144 Ser		tGc 509 tCc	
16		Cys 144 Tyr		tGc 509 tAc	
17		Cys 146 Arg		Tgc 514 Cgc	
18		Tyr 150 Cys		tAc 527 tGc	
19		Arg 153 Cys		Cgc 535 Tgc	
20	4	Cys 162 Ser		Tgc 562 Agc	
21		Arg 169 Cys		Cgc 583 Tgc	
22		Gly 171 Cys		Ggt 589 Tgt	
23		Cys 174 Phe		tGc 599 tTc	
24		Cys 174 Tyr		tGc 599 tAc	
25		Ser 180 Cys		tCc 617 tGc	
26		Arg 182 Cys		Cgc 622 Tgc	
27		Cys 183 Arg		Tgc 625 Cgc	
28		Cys 183 Ser		Tgc 625 Agc	
29		Cys 185 Arg		Tgt 631 Cgt	
30		Cys 185 Gly		Tgt 631 Ggt	
31		Cys 194 Arg		Tgt 658 Cgt	
32		Cys 194 Phe		tGt 659 tTt	
33		Cys 194 Tyr		tGt 659 tAt	
34	5	Cys 206 Tyr		tGc 695 tAc	
35		Arg 207 Cys		Cgt 697 Tgt	
36		Cys 212 Ser		Tgc 712 Agc	
37		Cys 222 Gly		Tgt 742 Ggt	
38		Cys 222 Tyr		tGt 743 tAt	
39		Cys 224 Tyr		tGt 749 tAt	
40	6	Cys 251 Arg	5	Tgc 829 Cgc	3.3
41	6	Tyr 258 Cys		tAt 851 tGt	
42	8	Arg 332 Cys	6	Cgc 1072 Tgc	1.7
43	10	Cys 428 Ser	8	tGt 1361 tCt	5.0
44	11	Cys 440 Gly		Tgc 1396 Ggc	
45		Arg 449 Cys		Cgc 1423 Tgc	
46	13	Cys 542 Tyr	11	tGt 1703 tAt	8.3
47	14	Arg 544 Cys		Cgc 1708 Tgc	
48		Arg 558 Cys		Cgc 1750 Tgc	
49		Arg 578 Cys		Cgc 1810 Tgc	

(continued)

Table 2.a. *Continued*

No	EGF Domain	Amino acid change	Exon	Notch 3 nucleotide change	% of mutations per exon*
50	15	Arg 607 Cys		Cgc 1897 Tgc	
51	18	Arg 728 Cys	14	Cgc 2260 Tgc	1.7
52	24	Gly 953 Cys	18	Ggc 2935 Tgc	5.0
53	25	Phe 984 Cys		tTc 3029 tGc	
54		Arg 985 Cys		Cgc 3031 Tgc	
55	26	Arg 1006 Cys	19	Cgc 3094 Tgc	6.7
56		Cys 1015 Arg		Tgc 3121 Cgc	
57		Tyr 1021 Cys		tAt 3141 tGt	
58		Arg 1031 Cys		Cgc 3169 Tgc	
59	27	Gly 1063 Cys	20		1.7
60	31	Arg 1231 Cys	22	Cgt 3769 Tgt	1.7
61	32	Cys 1261 Arg	23	Tgc 3859 Cgc	1.7
62	C-term	Ala 2223 Val	33	gCg 6746 gTg	Polymorphism**

Table 2.b. Other non-missense mutations

No	EGF Domain	Amino acid change	Exon	Notch 3 nucleotide change
1	2	In frame deletion of Gly114-Pro120 (gly, pro, asp, cys, ser, leu, pro	4	Deletion of G419 to G439 due to A to G transition in the 39 acceptor splice of exon 4
2		Asp80-Ser84, (asp, pro, cys, ser)		Deletion from 317–331
3	3	Arg153-Cys155, (arg, ser, cys)		Deletion from 537–545

Above mutation results compiled from following references and unpublished data: Ceroni et al., 2000; De Lange et al., 1999; Dichgans et al., 2000; Escary et al., 2000; Joutel et al., 1997, 2000b, 2001; Kalaria et al., unpublished data; Kotorii et al., 2001; *Low and Kalaria, unpublished observation; Markus et al., unpublished data; Meeks et al., 2001; Oberstein et al., 1999; Tuominen et al., 2001; Oliveri et al., 2001; Wang et al., 2000

* % of total of 60 different mutations in each exon. In addition to above at least 20 nucleotide substitutions not involving amino acid change (neutral mutation) have been reported. These occur in several different exons

A or *a* adenine; *Arg* arginine; *Asp* asparagine; *C* or *c* cytosine; *Cys* cysteine; *EGF* epidermal growth factor; *G* or *g* guanine; *Gly* glycine; *Phe* phenylalanine; *Ser* serine; *T* or *t* thymine; *Tyr* tyrosine

portions. The resulting segments are transported to the cell surface to form a heterodimeric receptor. The extracellular domain (NECD) may be shed with the ligand. The leucine zipper domain in NICD may regulate dimerisation. Protein interaction studies (Annaert and De Strooper, 1999) have suggested that PS1 or γ-secretase is required to release (by cleavage) NICD from the plasma membrane. Alternatively, PS1 may act by facilitating the activity of the protease responsible for cleavage. Other additional factors that likely influence signalling through these core elements and display molecular inter-

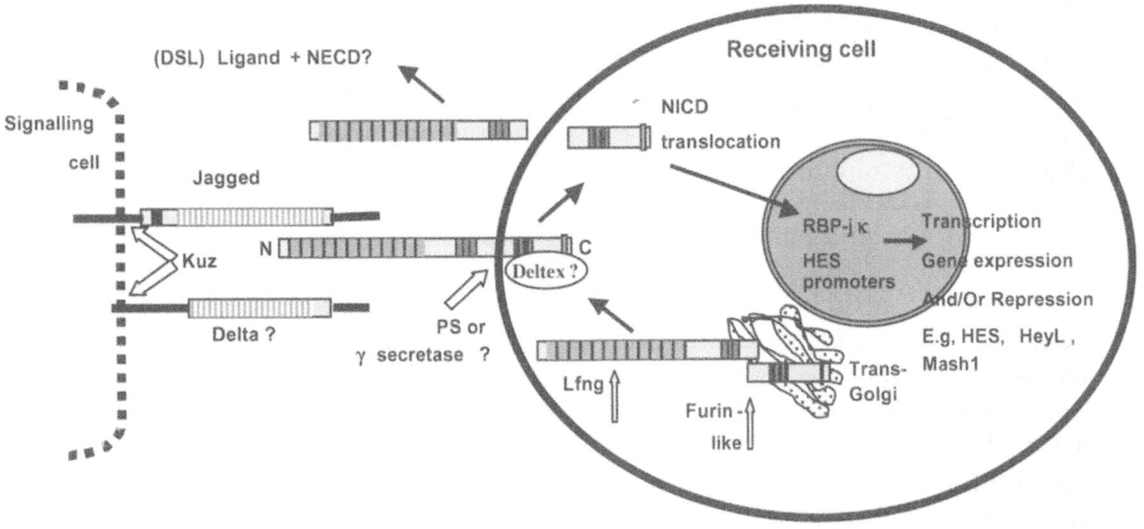

Fig. 4. A putative model for ligand-induced Notch signalling and processing of Notch 3 receptor. Notch 3 is expressed in precursor cells and undergoes post-translational modification within the transgolgi complex. These modifications include cleavage by a furin-like protease as well as glycosylation by Lunatic Fringe (Lfng). Processed Notch 3 receptor is transported to the plasma membrane as a heterodimeric receptor. Activation of Notch 3 signalling pathway occurs with the physical interaction of ligands expressed in signalling cell. Activation results in the cleavage of the Notch 3 receptor by a presenilin-1-dependent γ-secretase-like protease. The Notch 3 extracellular domain (NECD) is released into the extracellular matrix together with the extracellular domain of the DSL ligand, which may be cleaved by the metalloprotease, Kuzbanian (Kuz). The Notch 3 intracellular domain (NICD) translocates to the nucleus and interacts with transcription factors such as RBP-Jκ, Mastermind (MAML1), KyoT2, NF-κB. This results in either transcription activation or repression of the HES promoter (Beatus et al., 1999). The genes involved include the HES family, HeyL, Mash1 as well as E47 basic helix-loop-helix transcription factors. Activation of the Notch 3 signalling pathway within receiving cells remains undifferentiated at precursor stage. On the other hand, neighbouring cells that were not activated undergo lineage specific cell differentiation, which may depend on other extrinsic and intrinsic factors

actions are Kuzbanin, deltex, disheveled, and dab (Artavanis-Tsakonas et al., 1999).

The EGF domains and other conserved motifs including the cysteine-rich regions located immediately downstream may be negatively or positively regulated by various ligands at the cell surface. In the *drosophila* and *caenorhabditis elegans* expression of mutant forms lacking most or portions of the extracellular ligand-binding domain produces constitutively active proteins that function to inhibit normal cell-fate selection or differentiation. Therefore, the extracellular domain appears to inhibit the signalling activity of the intracellular domain, an inhibition that is normally relived through ligand binding (Fig. 4). That the 34 EGF repeats each bear about 40 residues suggests that the spatial arrangement of the repeats is also vital to its function of ligand binding and protein-protein interactions. By altering the quota of cysteine residues *Notch* 3 mutations may induce conformational changes at the DSL ligand-binding site of the receptor and disrupt the nuclear translocation of the intracellular carboxyl-terminal fragment. Alternatively, putative polymorphisms within the cdc 10/ankhyrin domains of *Notch* 3 could disrupt the nuclear binding of the intracellular portion to the RBP-jk and HES element(s) (Beatus et al., 1999). Aberrant Notch translocation may potentially disrupt interaction with other parallel signalling pathways like the Wnt (Dale, 1998).

CADASIL may be precipitated by either a gain-of-function (toxic) mutation or haploinsufficiency. The mutations may alter trafficking or processing of Notch 3 (Fig. 2). Alternatively, mutants may directly alter ligand binding through misfolding of the EGF region or promote oligomerisation of the receptor protein. Enrichment of Notch 3 protein and mRNA in vascular smooth muscle cells (Kalaria et al., 2000; Joutel et al., 2000a) and the evident vascular pathology suggest these primary targets are dependent on intact Notch 3 signalling (Fig. 4). Therefore, determining the role of Notch 3 function in the vasculature should elucidate how these mutations lead to the distinct pathology in the arterial vessels (Ruchoux and Murage, 1997). There can be little doubt that interest in this disorder in view of its link to the Notch signalling pathways implicated to interact with the Alzheimer's disease associated presenilins and their prototypes will bring new revelations (Ray et al., 1999). The elucidation of these issues and the vascular pathology will also provide further understanding of this devastating vascular disease afflicting the young and old that appears more common than the familial Alzheimer's disease. CADASIL also has important relevance to cerebrovascular disorders leading to stroke or dementing disorders in the elderly where ischaemic cerebral blood flow impinges on cognitive status.

Acknowledgments

We wish to thank N. Cookson and V. Pekovic for some of the analysis. We are also grateful to J. Hind for secretarial assistance. Our research programmes are supported by grants from Medical Research Council (UK), Alzheimer's Research Trust (UK), National Alzheimer's Association, USA (Zenith and IIRG Awards), and NINDS (NIH).

References

Adair JC, Hart BL, Kornfeld M, Graham GD, Swanda RM, Ptacek LJ, Davis LE (1998) Autosomal dominant cerebral arteriopathy: neuropsychiatric syndrome in a family. Neuropsychiatr Neuropsychol Behav Neurol 11: 31–39

Annaert W, De Strooper B (1999) Presenilins: molecular switches between proteolysis and signal transduction. TINS 22: 439–443

Artavanis-Tsakonas S, Rand MD, Lake RJ (1999) Notch signaling: cell fate control and signal integration in development. Science 284: 770–776

Beatus P, Lundkvist J, Oberg C, Lendahl U (1999) The notch intracellular domain represses Notch 1-mediated activation through hairy/Enhancer of split (HES) promoters. Development 126: 3925–3935

Bergmann M, Ebke M, Yuan Y, et al (1996) Cerebral autosomal dominant arteriopathy with subcortical infarcts and leukoencephalopathy (CADASIL): a morphological study of a German family. Acta Neuropathol 92: 341–350

Caronti B, Calandriello L, Francia A, et al (1998) Cerebral autosomal dominant arteriopathy with subcortical infarcts and leucoencephalopathy (CADASIL). Neuropathological and in vitro studies of abnormal elastogenesis. Acta Neurol Scand 98: 259–267

Ceroni M, Poloni TE, Tonietti S, Fabozzi D, Uggetti C, Frediani F, Simonetti F, Malaspina A, Alimonti D, Celano M, Ferrari M, Carrera P (2000) Migraine with aura and white matter abnormalities: Notch 3 mutation. Neurology 54: 1869–1871

Chabriat H, Vahedi K, Iba-Zizen MT, Joutel A, Nibbio A, Nagy TG, Krebs MO, Julien J, Dubois B, Ducrocq X, et al (1995) Clinical spectrum of CADASIL: a study of 7 families. Lancet 346: 934–939

Chabriat H, Levy C, Taillia H, et al (1998) Patterns of MRI lesions in CADASIL. Neurology 51: 452–457

Chuah TL, Tan SM, Flanagan S, Hyland V, Sullivan AA, Henderson R, MacMillan J, Lander C (2001) CADASIL (Cerebral Autosomal Dominant Arteriopathy with Subcortical Infarcts and Leucoencephalopathy): an Australian perspective. J Clin Neurosci 8: 404–406

Coulthard A, Blank SC, Bushby KMD, et al (1999) Distribution of cranial MRI abnormalities in patients with symptomatic and subclinical CADASIL. Br J Radiol 73: 256–265

Dale T (1998) Signal transduction by the Wnt family of ligands. Biochem J 329: 209–223

De Lange RPJ et al, Bolt J, Schanen C, et al (1999) Screening British CADASIL families for mutations in NOTCH3 gene. J Med Genet 37: 224–225

Desmond DW, Moroney JT, Lynch T, et al (1998) CADASIL in a North American family: clinical, pathologic, and radiologic findings. Neurology 51: 844–899

Desmond DW, Moroney JT, Lynch T, et al (1999) The natural history of CADASIL. A pooled analysis of previously published cases. Stroke 30: 1230–1233

Dichgans M, Mayer M, Uttner I, et al (1998) The phenotypic spectrum of CADASIL: clinical findings in 102 cases. Ann Neurol 44: 731–739

Dichgans M, Wick M, Gasser T (1999a) Cerebrospinal fluid findings in CADASIL. Neurology 39: 110–112

Dichgans M, Filippi M, Bruning R, et al (1999b) Quantitative MRI in CADASIL: correlation with disability and cognitive performance. Neurology 52: 1361–1367

Dichgans M, Ludwig H, Muller-Hocker J, Messerschmidt A, Gasser T (2000) Small in-frame deletions and missense mutations in CADASIL: 3D models predict misfolding of Notch 3 EGF-like repeat domains. Eur J Hum Genet 4: 280–285

Escary JL, Cecillon M, Maciazek J, Lathrop M, Tournier-Lasserve E, Joutel A (2000) Evaluation of DHPLC analysis in mutational scanning of Notch 3, a gene with a high G-C content. Hum Mutat 16: 518–526

Filley CM, Thompson LL, Sze CI, et al (1999) White matter dementia in CADASIL. J Neurol Sci 163: 163–167

Grand MG, Kaine J, Fulling K, Atkinson J, Dowton SB, Farber M, Craver J, Rice K (1988) Cerebroretinal vasculopathy. A new hereditary syndrome. Opthalmology 95: 649–658

Gutmann DH, Fischbeck KH, Sergott RC (1989) Hereditary retinal vasculopathy with cerebral white matter lesions. Am J Med Genet 34: 217–220

Hassan A, Markus H (2000) Genetics and ischaemic stroke. Brain 9: 1784–1812

Hedera P, Friedland RP (1997) CADASIL: study of two American families with predominant dementia. J Neurol Sci 146: 27–33

Ikeda H, Sasaki T, Yoshimoto T, Fukui M, Arinami T (1999) Mapping of a familial moyamoya disease gene to chromosome 3p24.2-p26. Am J Hum Genet 64: 533–537

Inoue TK, Ikezaki K, Sasazuki T, Matsushima T, Fukui M (2000) Linkage analysis of moyamoya disease on chromosome 6. J Child Neurol 15: 179–182

Jen J, Cohen AH, Yue Q, Stout JT, Vinters HV, Nelson S, Baloh RW (1997) Hereditary endotheliopathy with retinopathy, nephropathy, and stroke (HERNS). Neurology 49: 1322–1330

Joutel A, Corpechot C, Ducros A, Vahedi K, Chabriat H, Mouton P, Alamowitch S, Domenga V, Cecillion M, Marechal E, Maciazek J, Vayssiere C, Cruaud C, Cabanis EA, Ruchoux MM, Weissenbach J, Bach JF, Bousser MG, Tournier-Lasserve E (1996) Notch 3 mutations in CADASIL, a hereditary adult-onset condition causing stroke and dementia. Nature 383: 707–710

Joutel A, Vahedi K, Corpechot C, Troesch A, Chabriat H, Vayssiere C, Cruaud C, Maciazek J, Weissenbach J, Bousser MG, Bach JF, Tournier-Lasserve E (1997) Strong clustering and stereotyped nature of notch 3 mutations in CADASIL patients. Lancet 350: 1511–1515

Joutel A, Andreux F, Gaulis S, Domenga V, Cecillon M, Battail N, Piga N, Chapon F, Godfrain C, Tournier-Lasserve E (2000a) The ectodomain of the Notch 3 receptor accumulates within the cerebrovasculature of CADASIL patients. J Clin Invest 105: 597–605

Joutel A, Chabriat H, Vahedi K, Domenga V, Vayssiere C, Ruchoux MM, Lucas C, Leys D, Bousser MG, Tournier-Lasserve E (2000b) Splice site mutation causing a seven amino acid Notch 3 in-frame deletion in CADASIL. Neurology 9: 1874–1875

Joutel A, Dodick DD, Parisi JE, Cecillon M, Tournier-Lasserve E, Bousser MG (2000c) De novo mutation in the Notch 3 gene causing CADASIL. Ann Neurol 3: 388–391

Kalaria RN (1996) Cerebral vessels in ageing and Alzheimer's disease. Pharm Ther 72: 193–214

Kalaria RN (2001) Advances in molecular genetics and pathology of cerebrovascular disorders. Trends Neurosci 24: 392–400

Kalaria RN, Cookson NJ, Mizuno T, Oakley A, Singleton AB, Morris CM, De Lange RPJ, Burn DJ, St Clair D (2000) Microvascular pathology in familial multiinfarct dementia or CADASIL: implications for cerebral blood flow. Ischemic blood flow in the brain. Springer, Tokyo

Kalimo H, Haltia M (1997) Vascular diseases. In: Graham DI, Lantos PL (eds) Greenfield's neuropathology, 6th edn. Arnold, London, pp 315–396

Kalimo H, Viitanen M, Amberla K, Juvonen V, Marttila R, Poyhonen M, Rinne JO, Savontaus M, Tuisku S, Winblad B (1999) CADASIL: hereditary disease of the arteries causing brain infarcts and dementia. Neuropathol Appl Neurobiol 25: 257–265

Kamimura K, Takahashi K, Uyama E, Tokunaga M, Kotorii S, Uchino M, Tabira T (1999) Identification of a Notch 3 mutation in a Japanese CADASIL family. Cerebral autosomal dominant arteriopathy with subcortical infarcts and leukoencephalopathy. Alzheimer Dis Assoc Disord 13: 222–225

Kimble J, Simpson P (1997) The lin-12/notch signaling pathway and its regulation. Ann Rev Cell Dev Biol 13: 333–361

Kotorii S, Takahashi K, Kamimura K, Arima K, Yamada H, Uyama E, Uchino M, Suenaga A, Matsumoto M, Kuchel G, Rouleau GA, Tabira T (2001) Mutations of the Nootch 3 gene in non-caucasian patients with suspected CADASIL syndrome. Dement Geriatr Cogn Disord 12: 185–193

Lammie GA, Rakshi J, Rossor MN, et al (1995) Cerebral autosomal dominant arteriopathy with subcortical infarcts and leukoencephalopathy (CADASIL)-confirmation by cerebral biopsy in 2 cases. Clin Neuropathol 14: 201–206

Leys D, Erkinjuntti T, Desmond DW, Schmidt R, Englund E, Asquier F, Parnetti L, Ghika J, Kalaria RN, Chabriat H, Scheltens P, Bogousslavsky J (1999) Vascular dementia: the role of cerebral infarcts. Alzheimer Dis Assoc Disord 13: S38–48

Malandrini A, Carrera P, Ciacci G, et al (1997) Unusual clinical features and early brain MRI lesions in a family with cerebral autosomal dominant arteriopathy. Neurology 48: 1200–1203

Mellies JK, Baumer T, Muller JA, et al (1998) SPECT study of a German CADASIL family: a phenotype with migraine and progressive dementia only. Neurology 50: 1715–1721

Oberstein SA, Ferrari MD, Bakker E, et al (1999) Diagnostic Notch 3 sequence analysis in CADASIL: three new mutations in Dutch patients. Neurology 52: 1913–1915

Oliveri RL, Muglia M, De Stefano N, Mazzei R, Labate A, Conforti FL, Patitucci A, Gabriele AL, Tagarelli G, Magariello A, Zappia M, Gambardella A, Federico A, Quattrone A (2001) A novel mutation in the Notch 3 gene in an Italian family with cerebral autosomal dominant arteriopathy with subcortical infarcts and leukoencephalopathy: genetic and magnetic resonance spectroscopic findings. Arch Neurol 58: 1418–1422

Ray WJ, Yao M, Nowotny P, et al (1999) Evidence for a physical interaction between presenilin and Notch. Proc Natl Acad Sci USA 96: 3263–3268

Ruchoux MM, Maurage E (1997) Review on CADASIL. J Neuropathol Exp Neurol 56: 947–964

Salloway S, Hong J, et al (1998) CADASIL syndrome: a genetic form of vascular dementia. J Geriatr Psychiatry Neurol 11: 71–77

Shimizu K, Chiba S, Kumano K, Hosoya N, Takahashi T, Kanda Y, Hamada Y, Yazaki Y, Hirai H (1999) Mouse Jagged 1 physically interacts with Notch 2 and other Notch receptors. J Biol Chem 274: 32961–32969

Sourander P, Walinder J (1977) Hereditary multi-infarct dementia. Acta Neuropathol 39: 247–254

Stevens DL, Hewlett RH, Brownell B (1977) Chronic familial vascular encephalopathy. Lancet i: 1364–1365

Thomas NJ, Morris CM, Scaravilli F, Johanssen J, Rossor M, De Lange RPJ, St Clair D, Nicoll J, Blank SC, Coulthard A, Bushby KMD, Ince PG, Burn DJ, Kalaria RN (2000) Hereditary vascular dementia linked to Notch 3 mutations. Ann NY Acad Sci 903: 293–298

Tournier-Lasserve E (1999) CACNA1A mutations: hemiplegic migraine, episodic ataxia type 2, and the others. Neurology 53: 3–4

Trojano L, Ragno M, Manca A, et al (1998) A kindred affected by cerebral autosomal dominant arteriopathy with subcortical infarcts and leukoencephalopathy (CADASIL). A 2-year neuropsychological follow-up. J Neurol 245: 217–222

Tuominen S, Juvonen V, Amberla K, Jolma T, Rinne JO, Tuisku S, Kurki T, Marttila R, Poyhonen M, Savontaus ML, Viitanen M, Kalimo H (2001) Phenotype of a homozygous CADASIL patient in comparison to 9 age-matched heterozygous patients with the same R133C Notch 3 mutation. Stroke 32: 1767–1774

Utatsu Y, Utatsu Y, Takashima H, Michizono K, Kanda N, Endou K, Mitsuyama Y, Fujimoto T, Nagai M, Umehara F, Higuchi I, Arimura K, Nakagawa M, Osame M (1997) Autosomal dominant early onset dementia and leukoencephalopathy in a Japanese family: clinical neuroimaging and genetic studies. J Neurol Sci 147: 55–62

Wang T, Sharma SD, Fox N, Rossor M, Brown MJ, Sharma P (2000) Description of a simple test for CADASIL disease and determination of mutation frequencies in sporadic ischaemic stroke and dementia patients. J Neurol Neurosurg Psychiatry 69: 652–654

Weil S, Reifenberger G, Dudel C, Yousry TA, Schriever S, Noachtar S (1999) Cerebroretinal vasculopathy mimicking a brain tumor: a case of a rare hereditary syndrome. Neurology 53: 629–631

Weinmaster G (1997) The ins and outs of Notch signaling. Mol Cell Neurosci 9: 91–108

Yamauchi T, Tada M, Houkin K, Tanaka T, Nakamura Y, Kuroda S, Abe H, Inoue T, Ikezaki K, Matsushima T, Fukui M (2000) Linkage of familial moyamoya disease (spontaneous occlusion of the circle of Willis) to chromosome 17q25. Stroke 31: 930–935

Yousry TA, Seelos K, Mayer M, et al (1999) Characteristic MR lesion pattern and correlation of T1 and T2 lesion volume with neurolgic and neuropsychological find-

ings in cerebral autosomal dominant arteriopathy with subcortical infarcts and leukoencephalopathy (CADASIL). AJNR Am J Neuroradiol 20: 91–100
Zhang H, Sourander P, Olsson Y (1994) The microvascular changes in cases of hereditary multi-infarct disease of the brain. Acta Neuropathol 87: 317–324

Authors' address: Prof. R. N. Kalaria, Wolfson Research Centre, Institute for Ageing and Health, Newcastle General Hospital, Westgate Road, Newcastle upon Tyne NE4 6BE, United Kingdom, e-mail: r.n.kalaria@ncl.ac.uk

J Neural Transm (2002) [Suppl] 63: 91–109

Diagnosis and management of vascular cognitive impairment and dementia*

T. Erkinjuntti

Memory Research Unit, Department of Neurology, University of Helsinki, Finland

Summary. Vascular dementias (VaDs) are the second most common cause of dementia. Cerebrovascular disease (CVD) and stroke relates to high risk of cognitive impairment, but also relate to Alzheimer's disease (AD):

Vascular cognitive impairment (VCI) and dementias extend beyond the traditional multi-infarct dementia. Pathophysiology of VaD incorporates interactions between vascular etiologies (CVD and vascular risk-factors), changes in the brain (infarcts, white matter lesions, atrophy), host factors (age, education) and cognition.

Variation in defining the cognitive syndrome, in vascular etiologies, and allowable brain changes in current criteria have resulted in variable estimates of prevalence, of groups of subjects, and of the types and distribution of putative causal brain lesions.

Should new criteria be developed? Ideally in constructing new criteria the diagnostic elements should be tested with prospective studies with clinical-pathological correlation: replace dogma with data. Meanwhile focus on more homogenous subtypes of VaD, and on imaging criteria could be a solution.

Subcortical ischemic vascular disease and dementia (SIVD) incorporate small vessel disease as the chief vascular etiology, lacunar infarct and ischaemic white matter lesions as primary type of brain lesions, subcortical location as the primary location of lesions, and subcortical syndrome as the primary clinical manifestation. It incorporates two clinical entities "Binswanger's disease" and "the lacunar state".

AD with VaD (mixed dementia) has been underestimated as a prevalent cause in the older population. In addition to simple co-existence, VaD and AD have closer interaction: several vascular risk factors and vascular brain changes relate to clinical manifestation of AD, and they share also common pathogenetic mechanisms.

Vascular cognitive impairment (VCI) is a category aiming to replace the "Alzhemerized" dementia concept in the setting of CVD, and substitute it with a spectrum that includes subtle cognitive deficits of vascular origin, post-stroke dementia, and the complex group of the vascular dementias.

---

* A review based on a lecture given in the European Institute of Healthcare — CNS Symposium, December 1, 2001, Barcelona, Spain

As far there is no standard treatment for VaDs, and still little is known on the primary prevention (brain at risk for CVD) and secondary prevention (CVD brain at risk for VCI/VaD). There is no standard symptomatic treatment for VaD. Recently symptomatic cholinergic treatment has shown promise in AD with VaD, as well as probable VaD. Future focus should be directed to the distinct etiological and pathological factors: the vascular and the AD burden of the brain.

Introduction

Vascular dementias (VaDs) are the second most common causes of dementia (Rocca et al., 1991; Hebert and Brayne, 1995). Cerebrovascular disease (CVD) relates also to a high risk of cognitive impairment and dementia (Tatemichi et al., 1992, 1994). In addition, vascular factors such as coexisting stroke and white matter lesions (WMLs) relate also to Alzheimer's disease (AD) (Snowdon et al., 1997). Thus vascular causes is an important factor of cognitive impairment world-wide (Hachinski, 1992). Accordingly, early diagnosis of vascular factors affecting the brain, the vascular cognitive impairment (VCI) (Bowler and Hachinski, 1995) and VaDs is a challenge.

Background

As early as 1896 "arteriosclerotic dementia" (referring to VaD) was separated from "senile dementia" (referring to AD) (Berchtold and Cotman, 1998). Nevertheless, until the 1960s and 1970s cerebral atherosclerosis by causing chronic strangulation of blood supply to the brain, was thought to be the commonest cause of dementia, and AD was regarded as a rare cause affecting only younger patients. Tomlinson et al. (1970) reinvented AD as the more frequent cause of dementia than that of arteriosclerotic dementia. In 1979 Hachinski and colleagues used the term multi-infarct dementia (MID) to describe the mechanism by which they considered VaD was produced (Hachinski et al., 1974). As the pendulum swung in the direction of AD, vascular forms of dementia became relegated to a position of relative obscurity (Brust, 1988).

Despite until 1990's the concept of VaD has been that it is a dementia caused by small or large brain infarcts, that of MID (Hachinski et al., 1974; Erkinjuntti and Hachinski, 1993), VaD has come full circle with the resurgence of interest of the whole spectrum of vascular causes of cognitive impairment and dementia (Hachinski, 1990). This is supported by new data highlighting complex interactions between vascular aetiologies, changes in the brain, host factors and cognition (Chui, 1989; Tatemichi, 1990; Desmond, 1996; Pasquier and Leys, 1997; Skoog, 1998). Also reinvention of the heterogeneity of VaDs has fuelled the discussion. Further the facts that vascular factors relate and coexist with AD have strengthen interest on vascular burden of cognition (Skoog et al., 1999; Kalaria and Ballard, 1999).

Burden of the disease

Epidemiology of VaD has been affected by variations in the definition of the disorders, the clinical criteria used, and the clinical methods applied (Rocca et al., 1991; Lobo et al., 2000).

Prevalence. VaD is the second most common single cause of dementia accounting for 10 to 50% of the cases, depending on the geographic location, patient population and clinical methods used (Rocca et al., 1991; Hebert and Brayne, 1995; Lobo et al., 2000). Prevalence of VaD has been higher in China and Japan, compared to Europe and US. The prevalence of VaD has ranged from 1.2 to 4.2% in persons aged 65 years and older (Hebert and Brayne, 1995). In a recent European collaborative study using population-based studies of persons aged 65 years and older conducted in 1990s the age-standardized prevalence of dementia was 6.4% (all causes), 4.4% for AD and 1.6% for VaD (Lobo et al., 2000). In this study 15.8% of the cases had VaD and 53.7% AD. A large variation in VaD prevalence was seen across studies. The prevalence ranged from 0.0% to 0.8% at age 65 to 69 years, and from 2% to 8.3% at age 90 years and over in different studies. There was a difference in prevalence between men and women; under 85 years of age the prevalence of VaD was higher in men compared to women and thereafter the prevalence was higher in women. The pooled prevalence for the groups aged 65 to 69, 70 to 74, 75 to 79, 80 to 84, 85 to 89, and 90 years and older were 0.5%, 0.8%, 1.9%, 2.4%, 2.4%, and 3.0% in men. The corresponding figures for women were 0.1%, 0.6%, 0.9%, 2.3%, 3.5% and 5.8%, respectively.

Incidence. The incidence of VaD has varied between 6 to 12 cases per year in 1000 persons aged 70 years and older (Hebert and Brayne, 1995). The incidence of VaD increases with increasing age, without any substantial difference between men and women in a recent European collaborative study (Fratiglioni et al., 2000). In the European study the pooled incidence rate of VaD per 1000 person-years for the groups aged 65 to 69, 70 to 74, 75 to 79, 80 to 84, 85 to 89, and 90 years and older were 0.7%, 1.2%, 3.5%, 5.9%, 6.1%, and 8.1% (Fratiglioni et al., 2000).

Prognosis. The mean duration of any VaD is around five years (Hebert and Brayne, 1995), and their survival is less than for the general population or AD (Skoog et al., 1993; Mölsä et al., 1995). Also post-stroke dementia is an indepent predictor of mortality (Tatemichi et al., 1994). Detailed studies on the natural history of subcortical and cortical VaD are lacking, and little is known or can be predicted about the rate and pattern of cognitive decline, and prognosis VaD (Chui and Gonthier, 1999).

Post-stroke dementia. Recent studies has shown that CVD increases the risk of dementia. The frequency of dementia in a Japanese community-based study was 27.2% in patients with history of stroke and 3.4% in controls (Suzuki et al., 1991). In the New York study the prevalence of dementia three months after an ischemic stroke in patients aged 60 years or more was 26.3%, i.e. 9.4 fold higher than that of a stroke-free control group (Tatemichi et al., 1992). The risk was highest in the age-groups 70–79 years of age, with an Odds ratio (OR) of 31.2. In the Helsinki Stroke Aging Memory Study the frequency of DSM-III dementia 3 months post-stroke was 25% and the frequency was in the groups aged 55 to 64, 65 to 74, and 75 to 85 years 19%, 24%, and 32%, respectively (Pohjasvaara et al., 1997).

The frequencies of dementia reported after stroke in these studies are higher than those associated with any other known risk factor for dementia. In the New York study, stroke was the underlying cause of dementia in 56.1% of cases of dementia, while 36.4% are presumably due to the cumulative effects of stroke and AD (Tatemichi et al., 1992). In the Helsinki study the frequency of stroke-related dementia was 67.8% (Pohjasvaara et al., 1997).

Stroke patients have also an increased risk of dementia: one year after stroke the probability of new-onset dementia was 5.4% in patients over 60 years and 10.4% in patients over 90 years (Tatemichi, 1990). Four years after a first lacunar infarct, 23.1% of patients develop dementia i.e. 4 to 12 times more than controls (Loeb et al., 1992). Even after exclusion of patients who are demented 3 months after an ischemic stroke, the relative risk of dementia within 4 years is 5.5 (Tatemichi et al., 1994). In the community-based Rochester study, the standardized morbidity ratio for new-onset dementia was 8.6% for patients in the first year after stroke with the rate of new onset dementia doubling during the follow-up (Kokmen et al., 1996). The incidence rate of AD after stroke is also doubled, suggesting that stroke may induce an earlier expression of AD (Kokmen et al., 1996).

Pathophysiological heterogeneity

Vascular cognitive impairment (VCI) and dementia (VaD) is now seen to extend much beyond the traditional multi-infarct dementia (Chui, 1989; Erkinjuntti and Hachinski, 1993; Desmond, 1996; Erkinjunti, 1999). VaD as a clinical syndrome relates to different vascular mechanisms and changes in the brain, and has different causes and clinical manifestations. VaD is not only the traditional MID (Erkinjuntti and Hachinski, 1993; Chui, 1998). The pathophysiology of VaD incorporates interactions between vascular aetiologies (CVD and vascular risk-factors), changes in the brain (infarcts, WMLs, atrophy), host factors (age, education) and cognition (Chui, 1989; Tatemichi, 1990; Desmond, 1996; Pasquier and Leys, 1997; Skoog, 1998).

Etiologies of VaD include both CVDs and risk factors (Table 1). The main CVDs include large artery disease, cardiac embolic events, small vessel and hemodynamic mechanisms (Brun, 1994; Wallin and Blennow, 1994; Pantoni and Garcia, 1995; Amar and Wilcock, 1996; Erkinjuntti, 1996).

Riskfactors of VaDs (Table 1) include risk factors for CVD, stroke, WMLs, but, at the same time, also those of any cognitive decline and AD (Skoog, 1998).

Changes in the brain related to VaD include arterial territorial infarcts, distal field (watershed) infarcts, lacunar infarcts, ischaemic WMLs and incomplete ischaemic injury (Chui, 1989; Tatemichi, 1990; Brun, 1994; Erkinjuntti, 1996). In addition, both focal (around the ischaemic lesion) and remote (dis-

Table 1. Etiologies of vascular dementia

Cerebrovascular disorders
Large artery disease
Artery-to-artery embolism
Occlusion of an extra- or intracranial artery
Cardiac embolic events
Small vessel disease
Lacunar infarcts
Ischemic white matter lesions
Hemodynamic mechanisms
Specific arteriopathies
Hemorrhages
Intracranial hemorrhage
Subarachnoidal hemorrhage
Hematological factors
Venous diseases
Hereditary entities
Risk factors
Arterial hypertension
Atrial fibrillation
Cardiac abnormalities
Myocardial infarction
Coronary heart disease
Diabetes
Generalized atherosclerosis
Lipid abnormalities
Smoking
High age
Low education

connection, diaschisis) functional ischaemic changes relate to VaD (Mielke et al., 1992).

Relationship between vascular factors and cognition is essential, thus critical clinical issues include whether the identified vascular factors cause, compound or only coexist with the VaD syndrome (Erkinjuntti et al., 1988; Tatemichi et al., 1994), whether they contribute to the risk and clinical picture of AD (Pasquier and Leys, 1997; Snowdon et al., 1997), and which type, extent, side, site and tempo of vascular lesions in the brain relates to different types of VaD (Chui, 1989; Tatemichi, 1990; Desmond, 1996; Erkinjuntti, 1996).

Clinical criteria — definitional heterogeneity

Since 1970s several clinical criteria for VaD have been used (Erkinjuntti, 1994; Rockwood et al., 1994; Wetterling et al., 1996). The most widely used criteria for VaD include the DSM-IV (American Psychiatric Association, 1994), the ICD-10 (World Health Organization, 1993), the ADDTC criteria (Chui et al., 1992), and the NINDS-AIREN criteria (Roman et al., 1993).

The two cardinal elements implemented in the clinical criteria for VaD are (1) the definition of the cognitive syndrome of dementia (Erkinjuntti et al., 1997a), and (2) the definition of the vascular cause of the dementia (Wetterling et al., 1994; Erkinjuntti, 1994; Wetterling et al., 1996).

Variation in defining these two critical elements has namely caused that different definitions in use give different point prevalence estimates, identify different groups of subjects, and consequently also identify different types and distribution of brain lesions (Skoog et al., 1993; Wetterling et al., 1996; Pohjasvaara et al., 1997; Erkinjuntti et al., 1997a, 1999). Further, this heterogeneity may have been a factor for negative results in prior clinical trials on VaD (Inzitari et al., 2000).

All the clinical criteria used are consensus criteria, which are neither derived from prospective community based studies on vascular factors affecting the cognition, nor based on detailed natural histories (Chui et al., 1992; Roman et al., 1993; Erkinjuntti, 1994, 1997; Rockwood et al., 1994). All the cited criteria are mainly based on the ischemic infarct concept and designed to have high specificity, although they have been poorly implemented and validated (Rockwood et al., 1994; Erkinjuntti, 1997).

The *DSM-IV* definition for VaD requires focal neurological signs and symptoms **or** laboratory evidence of focal neurologic damage clinically judged to be related to the disturbance (American Psychiatric Association, 1994). The course is specified by sudden cognitive and functional losses. The DSM-IV criteria do not detail brain imaging requirements. The DSM-IV definition for VaD is reasonably broad and lack detailed clinical and radiological guidelines.

The *ICD-10* criteria (World Health Organization, 1993) require unequal distribution of cognitive deficits, focal signs as evidence of focal brain damage, and significant cerebrovascular disease judged to be etiologically related to the dementia. The criteria do not detail brain imaging requirements. The shortcoming of these criteria include lack of detailed guidelines (e.g. unequal cognitive deficits and neuroimaging), lack of etiological cues, and heterogeneity (Wetterling et al., 1994, 1996).

The *ADDTC* criteria are exclusively criteria for ischemic vascular dementia (IVD) (Chui et al., 1992). They require (1) evidence of two or more ischemic strokes by history, neurologic signs or neuroimaging studies (CT or T1-weighted MRI), or (2) in case of a single stroke a clearly documented temporal relationship (not specified in detail), and always a neuroradiological evidence of at least one infarct outside the cerebellum. Ischemic WMLs on CT or MRI do not qualify as brain imaging evidence of probable IVD, but may support a diagnosis of possible IVD. The criteria list features supporting the diagnosis, as well as a list of features casting doubt on a diagnosis of probable IVD.

The *NINDS-AIREN* research criteria for VaD (Roman et al., 1993) include dementia syndrome, cerebrovascular disease and a relationship between those. Cerebrovascular disease is defined by the presence of focal neurological sins and detailed brain imaging evidence of ischemic changes in the brain. A relationship between dementia and cerebrovascular disorder is based on the onset of dementia within 3 months following a recognised stroke, or on abrupt deterioration in cognitive functions or fluctuating, stepwise progression of cognitive deficits. The criteria include a list of features consistent with the diagnosis, as well as a list of features that make the diagnosis uncertain or unlikely. Also different levels of certainty of the clinical diagnosis (probable, possible, definite) are included. The inter-rater reliability of the NINDS-AIREN criteria has been shown to be moderate to substantial (kappa 0.46 to 0.72) (Lopez et al., 1994).

Comparison of clinical criteria. The current criteria for VaD are not interchangeable; the identify different numbers and cluster of patients labelled as VaD. The DSM-IV criteria are less restrictive compared to the ICD-10, the ADDTC and the NINDS-AIREN criteria (Verhey et al., 1996; Wetterling et al., 1996). The ADDTC criteria seem to be more sensitive and the NINDS-AIREN criteria more specific (Gold et al., 1997).

Heterogeneity of patients populations derived by using current criteria has raised a need for an updated systematisation. One suggestion has been that, by dividing VaD into subtypes, a more homogenous group of patients could be identified. A recent development are the new research criteria for subcortical VaD (Erkinjuntii et al., 2000).

Need of new classification and criteria

As reviewed, VaD is not a distinct disease, but a group of more ore less heterogeneous syndromes. An attempt to clarify this heterogeneity is to study possible clinical subtypes. The subtypes of VaD included in current classifications are the cortical VaD or MID, the subcortical ischemic VaD (SIVD) or the small vessel dementia, and the strategic infarct dementia (Erkinjuntti, 1987b; Roman et al., 1993; Brun, 1994; Cummings, 1994; Wallin and Blennow, 1994; Loeb and Meyer, 1996; Konno et al., 1997), and many include also the hypoperfusion dementia (Sulkava and Erkinjuntti, 1987; Roman et al., 1993; Brun, 1994; Cummings, 1994). Further subtypes suggested include hemorrhagic dementia, hereditary vascular dementia, and combined or mixed dementia (AD with CVD).

Cortical VaD (MID) relates to large vessel disease, cardiac embolic events and also hypoperfusion (Table 2). It shows predominantly cortical and cortico-subcortical arterial territorial and distal field (watershed) infarcts. Typical clinical features are lateralized sensorimotor changes and abrupt onset of cognitive impairment and aphasia (Erkinjuntti, 1987b; Erkinjuntti et al., 1988). In addition, some combination of different cortical neuropsychological syndromes has been suggested to be present in cortical VaD (Mahler and Cummings, 1991).

Strategic infarct dementia. Focal, often small, ischemic lesions involving specific sites critical for higher cortical functions have been classified separately. Of the cortical sites, the hippocampal formation, angluar gyrus and

Table 2. Vascular mechanisms and changes in the brain in main subtypes of vascular dementia

Vascular mechanisms	Changes in the brain
Cortical vascular dementia or multi-infarct dementia	
Large vessel disease	Arterial territorial infarct
Cardiac embolic events	Distal field (watershed) infarct
Hypoperfusion	
Subcortical ischemic vascular dementia or small vessel dementia	
Small vessel disease	Lacunar infarct
Hypoperfusion	Focal and diffuse white matter lesions
Incomplete ischemic injury	
Strategic infarct dementia	
Large vessel disease	Arterial territorial infarct
Cardiac embolic events	Distal field (watershed) infarct
Small vessel disease	Lacunar infarct
Hypoperfusion	Focal and diffuse white matter lesions

gyrus cinguli are examples. The subcortical sites include thalamus, fornix, basal forebrain, caudate, globus pallidus and the genu or anterior limb of the internal capsule (Tatemichi, 1990; Erkinjuntti and Hachinski, 1993; Erkinjuntti, 1996). Depending on the strategic location in question, the time-course and clinical features vary much.

Subcortical ischemic VaD (SIVD). This type of VaD incorporates two entities "the lacunar state" and "Binswanger disease". It relates to small vessel disease and is characterised by lacunar infarcts, focal and diffuse ischaemic WMLs, and incomplete ischemic injury (Roman, 1987; Erkinjuntti, 1987b; Mahler and Cummings, 1991).

Subcortical ischemic vascular disease and dementia (SIVD)

A more homogenous subtype of VaD for clinical trials, with a more predictable outcome, is the subcortical ischemic vascular disease and dementia (SIVD) (Erkinjuntti et al., 2000; Chui, 2001). The SIVD incorporate small vessel disease as the chief vascular etiology, lacunar infarct and ischaemic WMLs as primary type of brain lesions, subcortical location as the primary location of lesions, and subcortical syndrome as the primary clinical manifestation (Erkinjuntti et al., 2000).

Pathophysiology. The primary vascular mechanism in SIVD is the small vessel disease (Erkinjuntti and Pantoni, 2000; Pantoni and Lammie, 2001). The main risk factors of small vessel disease include age, arterial hypertension, diabetes, as well as genetic abnormality (e.g. CAA and CADACIL). The main types of SIVD small vessel change include arteriolosclerosis (deep perforating arterioles, 40–200 um, centrum semiovale and periventricular WM, leads to WMLs), lipohyalinosis (small perforating arteries and arterioles, 40–200 um, deep gray and white matter, lead to WMLs and lacunae) and intracerebral atherosclerosis (small perforating arteries, 200–850 u, deep gray matter, leads to lacunae) (Erkinjuntti and Pantoni, 2000; Pantoni and Lammie, 2001). Functionally the small vessel disease causes obliteration and occlusion of the vessel, increased tortuosity and coiling, increased resistance, decreased autoregulation, endothelia changes, change in the blood-brain barrier function and perivascular changes. Secondary SIVD risk factors include hemodynamic changes of systemic vascular, cardiac and carotid origin. These include e.g. arterial hypotension, blood pressure fluctuations, cardiac failure, cardiac arrhythmia and carotid stenosis. There are two pathways associated with small vessel disease (Chui, 2001). In the first pathway occlusion of a single arteriolar or arterial lumen leads to complete lacunar infarct. In the second pathway critical stenosis of multiple small vessels lead to hypoperfusion and incomplete infarcts. These complete infarcts relate to acute and severe ischemia leading to cystic necrosis with loss of all tissue elements. Incomplete infarction relate to more chronic, diffuse and less severe ischemia leading to selective loss of tissue elements in order of their selective vulnerability neuron > oligodendrocyte > myelinated axon > astrocyte > endothelial cell (Chui, 2001). Neuropathology of diffuse WMLs include araiosis, état crible, demyelination, axonal loss, changes in oligodendrocytes and glial cells, as well as noncavitated and cavitated small infarcts (Erkinjuntti et al., 1996; Erkinjuntti and Pantoni, 2000). Small vessel disease relates in addition to infarcts and WMLs, also to atrophy, as severity of cognitive impairment in SIVD correlate with medial temporal lobe atrophy, WMLs correlate with cortical atrophy (Chui, 2001) and WMLs correlate with medial temporal lobe atrophy (Erkinjuntti, personal communication 2001). SIVD incorporate two clinical entities "Binswanger's disease" and "the lacunar state" (Ishii et al., 1986; Babikian and Ropper, 1987; Roman, 1987).

Neuroimaging. The typical WMLs in SIVD include extending periventricular and deep WMLs affecting especially the genu or anterior limb of the internal capsule, anterior corona radiata and anterior centrum semiovale. The lacunes locate mainly in the caudate, globus pallidus, thalamus, internal capsule, corona radiata, frontal white matter. The brain imaging criteria of SIVD cover both cases having predominantly WMLs ("The Binswanger type"), and those with predominantly lacunar infarcts ("The lacunar state type") (Erkinjuntti et al., 2000). To include predominantly "white matter cases": extending periventricular and deep white matter lesions: extending caps (>10 mm as measured parallel to ventricle) or irregular halo (>10 mm broad, irregular margins and extending into deep white matter) *and* diffusely confluent hyperintensities (>25 mm, irregular shape) or extensive white matter change (diffuse hyperintensity without focal lesions), *and* lacune(s) in the deep grey matter. To include predominantly "lacunar cases": multiple lacunes (e.g. >5) in the deep gray matter *and* at least moderate white matter lesions: extending caps or irregular halo or diffusely confluent hyperintensities or extensive white matter changes.

Clinical features. The ischemic lesions in SIVD affect especially the prefrontal subcortical circuit (Cummings, 1993), which explains the main cognitive, behavioral and clinical neurological features.

Cognitive syndrome. The subcortical cognitive syndrome include both the executive dysfunction and memory deficit. Executive dysfunction includes impairment in goal formulation, initiation, planning, organizing, sequencing, executing, set-sifting and -maintenance, and abstracting. Memory deficit which can often be less severe, include impaired recall, relative intact recognition, less severe forgetting and benefit from cues. Behavioral and psychological symptoms include depression, personality change and psychomotor retardation.

Clinical syndrome. The two traditional clinical syndromes related to SIVD are that of "lacunar state" and "Binswanger syndrome" (Ishii et al., 1986; Babikian and Ropper, 1987; Roman, 1987; Chui, 2001). Clinical features of the lacunar syndrome include hemiparesis (pure sensory and motor, and other lacunar syndromes), pseudopulpar palsy and affect, small-stepped gait and urinary incontinence. The "Binswanger syndrome" include slowing of mental and motor processing, decreased initiative, depression, gait disturbance, and urinary incontinence. Early clinical features related to SIVD are episodes of mild upper motor signs (drift, reflex asymmetry, incordination), gait disorder (small-step gait or marche a petits-pa, magnetic, apraxic-ataxic or Parkinsonian gait), imbalance, urinary frequency and incontinence, exrapyramidal signs (hypokinesia and rigidity), as well as depression and mood changes.

Onset and cause. The onset is slow, less abrupt in 60% and gradual with or without acute deficits in 80% of the cases (Babikian and Ropper, 1987). This underlines the importance of neuroimaging criteria in the definitions of VaD.

Criteria. Clinical identification of patients with SIVD can be based on a modification of the NINDS-AIREN criteria for probable VaD (Roman et al., 1993; Erkinjuntti et al., 2000). The original criteria for NINDS-AIREN probable VaD also required a relationship between onset of dementia and cerebrovascular disease (CVD). In SIVD the onset is often more insidious, and a strong relationship already exist between the cognitive syndrome, brain imaging features, and evidence of CVD. Accordingly, this requirement was omitted from the research criteria of SIVD.

SIVD offers a solution to identify more homogenous and representative groups of patients, and is expected to show a more predictable clinical picture, natural history, outcomes, and treatment responses. Further empirical research is needed to define the syndrome and stages of SIVD, validate the brain imaging criteria for SIVD by clinical-pathological correlation, as well as characterize the natural history and outcomes of the syndrome. We have to go towards imaging (more sensitive and specific), towards ICVD (the disease), towards early and mild stages away from arbitary and late phenotype of dementia. Further we should find specific markers validated by clinical-pathological correlation for ICVD ad in order to independently quantitate both vascular and Alzheimer burden.

Clinical features of subcortical and cortical VaD

Early cognitive syndrome of subcortical VaD is characterized by (1) dysexecutive syndrome including slowed information processing, (2) memory deficit (may be mild), and (3) behavioral and psychological symptoms. The dysexecutive syndrome in subcortical VaD includes impairment in goal formulation, initiation, planning, organising, sequencing, executing, set-sifting and set-maintenance, as well as in abstracting (Mahler and Cummings, 1991; Cummings, 1994; Desmond et al., 1999). The memory deficit in subcortical VaD may be milder than e.g. in Alzheimer's disease, and is specified by impaired recall, relative intact recognition, less severe forgetting, and better benefit from cues (Desmond et al., 1999). Behavioural and psychological symptoms in subcortical VaD include in particulary depression, personality change, emotional lability and incontinence, as well as inertia, emotional bluntness and psychomotor retardation (Roman et al., 1993; Mahler and Cummings, 1991; Cummings, 1994).

Early cognitive syndrome of cortical VaD include some memory impairment (by definition) which may be mild, mostly some heteromodal cortical symptom(s) such as aphasia, apraxia, agnosia, visuospatial or constructional difficulty. In addition most patients have some degree of dysexecutive syndrome.

Clinical neurological findings especially early in the course of subcortical VaD include episodes of mild upper motor neuron signs (drift, reflex asymmetry, incordination), gait disorder (apractic-atactic or small-stepped), imbalance and falls, urinary frequency and incontinence, dysarthria, dysphagia, as well as extrapyramidal signs (hypokinesia, rigidity) (Ishii et al., 1986; Babikian and Ropper, 1987; Roman, 1987; Erkinjuntti, 1987b; Roman et al., 1993). However, often these focal neurological signs are subtle only (Fischer et al., 1990; Skoog, 1997a).

Patients with cortical VaD, having multiple cortico-subcortical infarcts often show field cut, lower facial weakness, lateralized sensimotor changes and gait impairment (hemiplegic, apractic-atactic) (Erkinjuntti, 1987b).

Onset and course. In subcortical VaD the onset is variable. For example in the series of Babikian and Ropper (1987) 60% of the patients had a slow, less abrupt onset, and only 30% an acute onset of cognitive symptoms. The course was gradual without (40%) and with (40%) acute deficits and acute stroke alone without progression in 13% (Babikian and Ropper, 1987).

Traditionally cortical VaD (MID) has been characterised by a relative abrupt onset (days to weeks), a step-wise deterioration (some recovery after worsening), and fluctuating course (e.g. difference between days) of cognitive functions (Roman, 1987; Erkinjuntti, 1987a; Chui et al., 1992; Roman et al., 1993; Fischer et al., 1990; Skoog, 1997a).

Alzheimer's disease with cerebrovascular disease

AD with CVD, the so-called mixed dementia syndrome may have been undepresented in our estimation of dementia subtypes (Rockwood et al., 1999). In addition to simple co-existence, VaD and AD seem to have closer interaction. Several vascular risk factors related to VaD have been shown also to be a risk factors of clinical AD (Skoog et al., 1999). In addition, infarcts and WMLs relate to a earlier clinical manifestation of AD (Snowdon et al., 1997). Further VaD and AD share also common pathogenetic mechanisms such as delayed neuronal death and apoptosis (Kalaria and Ballard, 1999). Overlap of these two mechanisms relate especially to the late-onset AD.

Clinical recognition of patients with mixed dementia or AD with CVD is problem. These patients have a clinical history and signs of CVD, being clinically more close to VaD. A solution could be to find reliable biological markers of clinical AD. Potential markers include e.g. early and significant medial temporal lobe atrophy on MRI, bilateral parietal hypoperfusion on SPECT, change in CSF beta amyloid and tau-protein, or e.g. presence of APO E 4 allele. On the other hand, in search of therapeutic approaches however, we may have to choose a new focus. Instead of being prisons of old diagnostic dichotomies (pure AD vs. pure VaD), we should change the focus on etiopathogenetic factors, measure both the vascular burden of the brain, as well as the Alzheimer burden of the brain, and their consequences.

Differential diagnosis

Differential diagnosis of VaDs include a number of conditions including normal pressure hydrocephalus, frontal lobe tumor, Lewy body dementia, frontotemporal degenerations, Parkinson's disease with dementia, progressive supranuclear palsy, and multisysten atrophy. Here we focus on the differential diagnosis between VaD and AD, as well as mention the problem of mixed dementia.

Alzheimers disease. AD has typical neuropathological stages (transentorhinal, limbic and neocortical) corresponding to clinical stages (preclinical, early and mild dementia) (Braak and Braak, 1991). Accordingly, AD is a typical stage concurrent disorder, progressing from mild cognitive impairment (MCI), to early pre-dementia AD and then to stages of AD dementia (Petersen, 1995), and is not a diagnosis of exclusion.

Taken the clinical series on differential diagnosis between AD and VaD, the main limitations have included (1) definition of the cognitive syndrome, the dementia syndrome, (2) definition of the cause/etiology of the dementia syndrome, and (3) heterogeneity of patient populations, especially that of VaDs.

The traditional concept of dementia has been based on the typical clinical features of AD (McKhann et al., 1984; Erkinjuntti et al., 1997b). The definition, has been the prison of AD, as the focus has been early episodic memory impairment, more or less global cognitive syndrome, with progressive course,

Table 3. Differential diagnosis between vascular dementia and Alzheimer's disease

Vacsular dementia	Alzheimer's disease
Early cognitive syndrome	
DYSEXECUTIVE SYNDROME	IMPAIRED EPISODIC MEMORY
Impaired planning, sequencing, Speed of processing	Ineffective learning, Increased forgetting, Impaired regognition, Poor response to Cues, Intrusion errors
MEMORY IMPAIRMENT (often mild)	Ineffective learning, Less forgetting
Preserved recognition, Good response Cues, Perseveration	
CORTICAL SYMTOM (S) (variable)	ANOMIA (mild)
Aphasia, apraxia, agnosia, visuospatial and constructive difficulty	VISUOSPATIAL IMPAIMRNT (mild)
Early clinical features	
Mild UMN signs (motor deficit, decreased coordination, brisk tendon reflexes, Babinski's sign)	Absence of focal neurological sings Dysthymia, mild depression
Gait disorder, Imbalance	
Urine frequency	
Dysarthria	
Mood changes, Depression	
Onset	
Variable: Relative abrupt, Insidious	Insidious
Clinical course	
Variable: Fluctuating, Stepwise, Progressive, Stable	Progressive May have plateaus

and major restrictions of ADLs. These are features different from that in early cases of VaD, and these criteria merely detect an end stage of VaD. One consequence has been, that different definitions of dementia syndrome, identify different groups of subjects both in epidemiological studies (Erkinjuntti et al., 1997b) and clinical post-stroke series (Pohjasvaara et al., 1997).

The most widely used definition of the cause of the cognitive syndrome includes the NINDS-AIREN for probable VaD (Roman et al., 1993) and the NINCDS-ADRDA for probable AD (McKhann et al., 1984). These criteria define a stereotyped set of patient groups (Table 3): probable VaD characterized by abrupt onset, or fluctuating and stepwise course with clinical signs of CVD and relevant CVD on brain imaging. In the contrary AD is characterized by insidious onset, progressive course, without clinical signs of CVD and without signs of CVD in brain imaging. Accordingly, in typical cases the differentiation between probable VaD and AD using common clinical tools is direct (Erkinjuntti et al., 1988).

Hachinski Ischemic Score has been widely used to differentiate patients with VaD and AD (Hachinski et al., 1975). In most clinical series the majority of the items differentiate VaD from probable AD — as a matter of fact this is based on the clinical definitions used. However, in a large neuropathologically confirmed series by Moroney et al. (1997) the independent correlates of VaD were stepwise deterioration (OR 6.1), fluctuating course (OR 7.6), history of hypertension (OR 4.3), history of stroke (OR 4.3) and history of focal neurological symptoms (OR 4.4).

AD and CVD (Mixed dementia). The issue of mixed dementia is a challenge. Increasing evidence shows that different vascular factors are related to AD, and frequently CVD coexist with AD (Skoog et al., 1999; Kalaria and Ballard, 1999). This overlap is increasingly important in older populations. Clinical recognition of patients with mixed dementia or AD with CVD, however, is a problem. As detailed in the neuropathological series of Moroney et al. (1997) these patients have a clinical history and signs of CVD, being clinically more close to VaD. In fact, in this series fluctuating course (OR 0.2) and history of strokes (OR 0.1) were the only items differentiating AD from the mixed cases.

Problematic clinical examamples include stroke unmasking AD in patients with post-stroke dementia, insidious onset and/or slow progressive course in VaD patients, and cases where difficulty exists in assessing the role of less extensive WMLs or of distinct infarcts on neuroimaging. This clinical challenge may be solved when a sensitive and specific ante-mortal marker for AD is available, and the distinction between AD and VaD could be supported by more detailed knowledge on which site, type and extent of ischaemic brain changes are critical for VaD and which extent and type of medial temporal lobe atrophy specifies AD.

Prevention and therapy

Primary prevention is aiming to reduce the incidence of disease by eliminating the causes or main risk factors (Last, 1988; Skoog, 1999). Thus in relation to vascular dementia the targets are risk factors of CVD and cognitive impairment, but also putative protective factors (Skoog, 1998). Factors include arterial hypertension, atrial fibrillation, myocardial infarction, coronary heart disease, diabetes, generalized atherosclerosis, lipid abnormalities and smoking. Putative protective factors are estrogen, anti-inflammatory agents and antioxidants (Mortel and Meyer, 1995). Knowledge of the effects of primary prevention of VaD is still scanty (Skoog, 1997b, 1998).

Secondary prevention is aiming to prevent the disease from progressing into a more serious outcome by means of early detection followed by treatment (Skoog, 1999). Actions in the population at risk of VCI and VaDs include (1) early diagnosis and treatment of acute stroke in order to limit the extent of ischaemic brain changes and to promote recovery, (2) prevention of stroke recurrence according the type of stroke, and (3) intensifying treatment of risk factors. Selection of treatment is guided by the etiology of CVD such as large artery disease (e.g. aspirin, dipyridamole, klopidogrel, carotid endarterectomy), cardiac embolic events (e.g. anticoagulation, aspirin), small-vessel disease (e.g. antiplatelet therapy as in large vessel disease), and hemodynamic mechanisms (e.g. control of hypotension and cardiac arrhythmias)

(Amar and Wilcock, 1996; Konno et al., 1997; Erkinjuntti, 1997). Hypoxic ischemic events (cardiac arrhythmias, congestive heart failure, myocardial infarction, seizures, pneumonia) are an important risk factor for incident dementia in patients with stroke and should be taken into account in the secondary prevention of VaD (Moroney et al., 1996).

Detailed knowledge of effects of secondary prevention directed towards the vascular component of VaD is still scanty. In small series of patients with established VaD control of high arterial blood pressure (Meyer et al., 1986), cessation of smoking (Meyer et al., 1986) and use of aspirin (Meyer et al., 1989) has improved or stabilised cognition. It has been suggested that lowering of plasma viscosity could also have an effect in VaD (Lechner, 1998). Further, absence of progressive cognitive decline in patients receiving placebo in symptomatic treatment trials of VaD may also reflect an effect of intensified risk factor control (Rother et al., 1998).

Symptomatic treatment or tertiary prevention. A number of drugs have been studied for symptomatic treatment of VaD including cerebro- and vasoactive drugs, nootropics and some calcium antagonists, but these studies have largely shown negative results (Knezevic et al., 1996). The studies have mostly had small numbers, short treatment periods, variations in diagnostic criteria and tools, often included mixed populations, and have had variations in the application of clinical endpoints (Erkinjunti, 1999). Recently both nimodipine (Pantoni et al., 1996), memantine (Görtelmeyer and Erbler, 1992), and propentofylline (Rother et al., 1998) have raised expectations in the symptomatic treatment of VaD. It is possible that the symptomatic treatment with acetylcholinesterase inhibitors, may prove effective also on the cognitive symptoms of VaD. First ever results in this area have been encouraging (Erkinjunti et al., 2001). Still at present there is no accepted standard symptomatic treatment of VaDs (Doody et al., 2001).

References

Amar K, Wilcock G (1996) Vascular dementia [Review] [65 refs]. BMJ 312: 227–231

American Psychiatric Association (1994) Diagnostic and statistical manual of mental disorders, 4th ed. American Psychiatric Association, Washington, DC

Babikian V, Ropper AH (1987) Binswanger's disease: a review. Stroke 18: 2–12

Berchtold NC, Cotman CW (1998) Evolution in the conceptualization of dementia and Alzheimer's disease: Greco Roman period to the 1960s. Neurobiol Aging 19: 173–189

Bowler JV, Hachinski V (1995) Vascular cognitive impairment: a new approach to vascular dementia. [Review] [75 refs]. Baillieres Clin Neurol 4: 357–376

Braak H, Braak E (1991) Neuropathological stageing of Alzheimer-related changes. Acta Neuropathol (Berl) 82: 239–259

Brun A (1994) Pathology and pathophysiology of cerebrovascular dementia: pure subgroups of obstructive and hypoperfusive etiology. Dementia 5: 145–147

Brust JC (1988) Vascular dementia is overdiagnosed [Review] [76 refs]. Arch Neurol 45: 799–801

Chui HC (1989) Dementia: a review emphasizing clinicopathologic correlation nd brain-behavior relationships. Arch Neurol 46: 806–814

Chui HC (1998) Rethinking vascular dementia: moving from myth to mechanism. In: Growdon JH, Rossor MN (eds) The dementias. Butterworth-Heinemann, Boston, pp 377–401
Chui HC (2001) Vascular dementia, a new beginning. Shifting focus from clinical phenotype to ischemic brain injury. Neuroloci clinics 18: 951–977
Chui HC, Gonthier R (1999) Natural history of vascular dementia. Alzheimer Dis Assoc Disord
Chui HC, Victoroff JI, Margolin D, Jagust W, Shankle R, Katzman R (1992) Criteria for the diagnosis of ischemic vascular dementia proposed by the State of California Alzheimer's Disease Diagnostic and Treatment Centers [see comments]. Neurology 42: 473–480
Cummings JL (1993) Fronto-subcortical circuits and human behavior. Arch Neurol 50: 873–880
Cummings JL (1994) Vascular subcortical dementias: clinical aspects [Review] [25 refs]. Dementia 5: 177–180
Desmond DW (1996) Vascular dementia: a construct in evolution [Review] [215 refs]. Cerebrovasc Brain Metab Rev 8: 296–325
Desmond DW, Erkinjuntti T, Sano M et al (1999) The cognitive syndrome of vascular dementia: implications for clinical trials. Alzheimer Dis Assoc Disord
Doody RS, Stevens JC, Beck C et al (2001) Practice parameter: Management of dementia (an evidence-based review). Report of the Quality Standards Subcommittee of the American Academy of Neurology. Neurology 56: 1154–1166
Erkinjuntti T (1987a) Differential diagnosis between Alzheimer's disease and ascular dementia: evaluation of common clinical methods. Acta Neurol Scand 76: 433–442
Erkinjuntti T (1987b) Types of multi-infarct dementia. Acta Neurol Scand 75: 391–399
Erkinjuntti T (1994) Clinical criteria for vascular dementia: the NINDS-AIREN criteria. Dementia 5: 189–192
Erkinjuntti T (1996) Clinicopathological study of vascular dementia. In: Prohovnik I, Wade J, Knezevic S, Tatemichi TK, Erkinjuntii T (eds) Vascular dementia. Current concepts. John Wiley & Sons, Chichester, pp 73–112
Erkinjuntti T (1997) Vascular dementia: challenge of clinical diagnosis. Int Psychogeriatr 9: 51–58
Erkinjunti T (1999) Cerebrovascular dementia: a quide to diagnosis and treatment. CNS Drugs
Erkinjuntti T, Hachinski VC (1993) Rethinking vascular dementia. Cerebrovasc Dis 3: 3–23
Erkinjuntti T, Pantoni L (2002) Subcortical vascular dementia. In: Gauthier S, Cummings JL (eds) Alzheimer's diasease and related disorders annual. Martin Dunitz, London, pp 101–133
Erkinjuntti T, Haltia M, Palo J, Sulkava R, Paetau A (1988) Accuracy of the clinical diagnosis of vascular dementia: a rospective clinical and post-mortem neuropathological study. J Neurol Neurosurg Psychiatry 51: 1037–1044
Erkinjuntti T, Benavente O, Eliasziw M et al (1996) Diffuse vacuolization (spongiosis) and arteriolosclerosis in the frontal white matter occurs in vascular dementia. Arch Neurol 53: 325–332
Erkinjuntti T, Ostbye T, Steenhuis R, Hachinski V (1997a) The effect of different diagnostic criteria on the prevalence of dementia. N Engl J Med 337: 1667–1674
Erkinjuntti T, Ostbye T, Steenhuis R, Hachinski V (1997b) The effect of different diagnostic criteria on the prevalence of dementia. N Engl J Med 337: 1667–1674
Erkinjuntti T, Bowler JV, DeCarli C et al (1999) Imaging of static brain lesions in vascular dementia: implications for clinical trials. Alzheimer Dis Assoc Disord 13: S81–S90
Erkinjuntti T, Inzitari D, Pantoni L et al (2000) Research criteria for subcortical vascular dementia in clinical trials. J Neural Transm 59: 23–30

Erkinjunti T, Kurz A, Gauthier S, Bullock R, Lilienfeld S, ChandrasekharRao VD (2001) Galantamine is efficacious in probable vascular dementia and Alzheimer's disease combined with cerebrovascular disease. J Am Ger Soc (in press)

Fischer P, Gatterer G, Marterer A, Simanyi M, Danielczyk W (1990) Course characteristics in the differentiation of dementia of the Alzheimer type and multi-infarct dementia. Acta Psychiatr Scand 81: 551–553

Fratiglioni L, Launer LJ, Andersen K et al (2000) Incidence of dementia and major subtypes in Europe: a collaborative study of population-based cohorts. Neurology 54: S10–S15

Gold G, Giannakopoulos P, Montes-Paixao JC et al (1997) Sensitivity and specificity of newly proposed clinical criteria for possible vascular dementia. Neurology 49: 690–694

Görtelmeyer R, Erbler H (1992) Memantine in treatment of mild to moderate dementia syndrome. Drug Res 42: 904–912

Hachinski VC (1990) The decline and resurgence of vascular dementia [Review] [41 refs]. CMAJ 142: 107–111

Hachinski V (1992) Preventable senility: a call for action against the vascular dementias [see comments] [Review] [33 refs]. J Am Ger Soc 340: 645–648

Hachinski VC, Lassen NA, Marshall J (1974) Multi-infarct dementia. A cause of mental deterioration in he elderly. J Am Ger Soc ii: 207–210

Hachinski VC, Iliff LD, Zilhka E et al (1975) Cerebral blood flow in dementia. Arch Neurol 32: 632–637

Hebert R, Brayne C (1995) Epidemiology of vascular dementia [Review] [75 refs]. Neuroepidemiology 14: 240–257

Inzitari D, Erkinjuntti T, Wallin A, del Ser T, Romanelli M, Pantoni L (2000) Subcortical vascular dementia as a specific target for clinical trials. Ann NY Acad Sci 903: 510–521

Ishii N, Nishihara Y, Imamura T (1986) Why do frontal lobe symptoms predominate in vascular dementia with lacunes? Neurology 36: 340–345

Kalaria RN, Ballard C (1999) Overlap between pathology of Alzheimer disease and vascular dementia. Alzheimer Dis Assoc Disord 13: S115–S123

Knezevic S, Labs KH, Kittner B, Rössner M, Rother M (1996) The treatment of vascular dementia: problems and prospects. In: Prohovnik I, Wade J, Knesevich J, Tatemichi TK, Erkinjunti T (eds) Vascular dementia. Current concepts. John Wiley & Sons, Chichester, pp 301–312

Kokmen E, Whisnant JP, O'Fallon WN, Chu CP, Beard CM (1996) Dementia after ischemic stroke: a population-based study in Rochester, Minnesota (1960–1984). Neurology 46: 154–159

Konno S, Meyer JS, Terayama Y, Margishvili GM, Mortel KF (1997) Classification, diagnosis and treatment of vascular dementia [Review] [83 refs]. Drugs & Aging 11: 361–373

Last JM (1988) A dictionary of epidemiology, 2nd edn. Oxford University Press, New York

Lechner H (1998) Status of treatment of vascular dementia [Review] [19 refs]. Neuroepidemiology 17: 10–13

Lobo A, Launer LJ, Fratiglioni L et al (2000) Prevalence of dementia and major subtypes in Europe: a collaborative study of population-based cohorts. Neurology 54: S4–S9

Loeb C, Meyer JS (1996) Vascular dementia: still a debatable entity? [Review] [50 refs]. J Neurol Sci 143: 31–40

Loeb C, Gandolfo C, Croce R, Conti M (1992) Dementia associated with lacunar infarction. Stroke 23: 1225–1229

Lopez OL, Larumbe MR, Becker JT et al (1994) Reliability of NINDS-AIREN clinical criteria for the diagnosis of vascular dementia [see comments]. Neurology 44: 1240–1245

Mahler ME, Cummings JL (1991) The behavioural neurology of multi-infarct dementia. Alzheimer Dis Assoc Disord 5: 122–130
McKhann G, Drachman D, Folstein M, Katzman R, Price D, Stadlan EM (1984) Clinical diagnosis of Alzheimer's disease: report of the NINCDS-ADRDA Work Group under the auspices of Department of Health and Human Services Task Force on Alzheimer's Disease. Neurology 34: 939–944
Meyer JS, Judd BW, Tawaklna T, Rogers RL, Mortel KF (1986) Improved cognition after control of risk factors for multi-infarct dementia. JAMA 256: 2203–2209
Meyer JS, Rogers RL, McClintic K, Mortel KF, Lotfi J (1989) Randomized clinical trial of daily aspirin therapy in multi-infarct dementia. A pilot study. J Am Geriatr Soc 37: 549–555
Mielke R, Herholz K, Grond M, Kessler J, Heiss WD (1992) Severity of vascular dementia is related to volume of metabolically impaired tissue. Arch Neurol 49: 909–913
Moroney JT, Bagiella E, Desmond DW, Paik MC, Stern Y, Tatemichi TK (1996) Risk factors for incident dementia after stroke. Role of hypoxic and ischemic disorders. Stroke 27: 1283–1289
Moroney JT, Bagiella E, Desmond DW et al (1997) Meta-analysis of the Hachinski Ischemic Score in pathologically verified dementias. Neurology 49: 1096–1105
Mortel KF, Meyer JS (1995) Lack of postmenopausal estrogen replacement therapy and the risk of dementia. J Neuropsychiatr Clin Neurosci 7: 334–337
Mölsä PK, Marttila RJ, Rinne UK (1995) Long-term survival and predictors of mortality in Alzheimer's disease and multi-infarct dementia. Acta Neurol Scand 91: 159–164
Pantoni L, Garcia JH (1995) The significance of cerebral white matter abnormalities 100 years after Binswanger's report. A review [Review] [164 refs]. Stroke 26: 1293–1301
Pantoni L, Lammie A (2002) Cerebral small vessel disease: pathological and pathophysiological aspects in relation to vascular cognitive impairment. In: Erkinjunti T, Gauthier S (eds) Vascular cognitive impairment. Martin Dunitz, London
Pantoni L, Carosi M, Amigoni S, Mascalchi M, Inzitari D (1996) A preliminary open trial with nimodipine in patients with cognitive impairment and leukoaraiosis. Clin Neuropharmacol 19: 497–506
Pasquier F, Leys D (1997) Why are stroke patients prone to develop dementia? [Review] [94 refs]. J Neurol 244: 135–142
Petersen RC (1995) Normal aging, mild cognitive impairment, and early Alzheimer's disease. The Neurologist 1: 326–344
Pohjasvaara T, Erkinjuntti T, Vataja R, Kaste M (1997) Dementia three months after stroke. Baseline frequency and effect of different definitions of dementia in the Helsinki Stroke Aging Memory Study (SAM) cohort. Stroke 28: 785–792
Rocca WA, Hofman A, Brayne C et al (1991) The prevalence of vascular dementia in Europe: facts and fragments from 1980–1990 studies. EURODEM-Prevalence Research Group. Ann Neurol 30: 817–824
Rockwood K, Parhad I, Hachinski V et al (1994) Diagnosis of vascular dementia: Consortium of Canadian Centres for Clinical Cognitive Research concensus statement [Review] [60 refs]. Can J Neurol Sci 21: 358–364
Rockwood K, Bowler J, Erkinjunti T, Hachinski V, Wallin A (1999) Subtypes of vascular dementia. Alzheimer Dis Assoc Disord 13: S59–S64
Roman GC (1987) Senile dementia of the Binswanger type. A vascular form of dementia in the elderly. JAMA 258: 1782–1788
Roman GC, Tatemichi TK, Erkinjuntti T et al (1993) Vascular dementia: diagnostic criteria for reserach studies. Report of the NINDS-AIREN International Work Group. Neurology 43: 250–260
Rother M, Erkinjuntti T, Roessner M, Kittner B, Marcusson J, Karlsson I (1998) Propentofylline in the treatment of Alzheimer's disease and vascular dementia. Dementia Geriatr Cogn Disord 9: 36–43

Skoog I (1997) Blood pressure and dementia. In: Hansson L, Birkenhäger WH (eds) Handbook of hypertension, vol 18. Assessment of hypertensive organ damage. Elsevier Science BV, Amsterdam, pp 303–331

Skoog I (1997b) The relationship between blood pressure and dementia: a review [Review] [139 refs]. Biomed Pharmacother 51: 367–375

Skoog I (1998) Status of risk factors for vascular dementia [Review] [89 refs]. Neuroepidemiology 17: 2–9

Skoog I, Nilsson L, Palmertz B, Andreasson L-A, Svanborg A (1993) A population-based study on dementia in 85-year-olds. N Engl J Med 328: 153–158

Skoog I, Kalaria RN, Breteler MMB (1999) Vascular factors and Alzheimer's disease. Alzheimer Dis Assoc Disord 13: S106–S114

Snowdon DA, Greiner LH, Mortimer JA, Riley KP, Greiner PA, Markesbery WR (1997) Brain infarction and the clinical expression of Alzheimer disease. The Nun Study [see comments]. JAMA 277: 813–817

Sulkava R, Erkinjuntti T (1987) Vascular dementia due to cardiac arrhythmias and systemic ypotension. Acta Neurol Scand 76: 123–128

Suzuki K, Kutsuzawa T, Nakajima K, Hatano S (1991) Epidemiology of vascular dementia and stroke in Akita, Japan. In: Hartmann A, Kuchinsky W, Hoyer S (eds) Cerebral ischemia and dementia. Springer, New York, pp 16–24

Tatemichi TK (1990) How acute brain failure becomes chronic. A view of the echanisms and syndromes of dementia related to stroke. Neurology 40: 1652–1659

Tatemichi TK, Desmond DW, Mayeux R et al (1992) Dementia after stroke: baseline frequency, risks, and clinical features in a hospitalized cohort. Neurology 42: 1185–1193

Tatemichi TK, Paik M, Bagiella E, Desmond DW, Pirro M, Hanzawa LK (1994) Dementia after stroke is a predictor of long-term survival. Stroke 25: 1915–1919

Tatemichi TK, Paik M, Bagiella E et al (1994) Risk of dementia after stroke in a hospitalized cohort: results of a longitudinal study. Neurology 44: 1885–1891

Tomlinson BE, Blessed G, Roth M (1970) Observations on the brains of demented old people. J Neurol Sci 11: 205–242

Verhey FR, Lodder J, Rozendaal N, Jolles J (1996) Comparison of seven sets of criteria used for the diagnosis of vascular dementia. Neuroepidemiology 15: 166–172

Wallin A, Blennow K (1994) The clinical diagnosis of vascular dementia [Review] [11 refs]. Dementia 5: 181–184

Wetterling T, Kanitz RD, Borgis KJ (1994) The ICD-10 criteria for vascular dementia. Dementia 5: 185–188

Wetterling T, Kanitz RD, Borgis KJ (1996) Comparison of different diagnostic criteria for vascular dementia (ADDTC, DSM-IV, ICD-10, NINDS-AIREN). Stroke 27: 30–36

World Health Organization (1993) ICD-10 Classification of mental and behavioural disorders: diagnostic criteria for research. WHO, Geneva

Author's address: Dr. T. Erkinjuntti, Memory Research Unit, Department of Neurology, University of Helsinki, P.O. Box 300, 00029 HUS, Helsinki, Finland, e-mail: timo.erkinjuntti@hu

J Neural Transm (2002) [Suppl] 63: 111–127

The genetics of migraine: implication for treatment approaches

M. D. Ferrari[1] and **J. Haan**[1,2]

[1] Department of Neurolgy, Leiden University Medical Center, Leiden, and
[2] Department of Neurology, Rijnland Hospital Leiderdorp, The Netherlands

Summary. Migraine is a paroxysmal neurological disorder affecting up to 12% of males and 24% of females in the general population, demonstrated to have a strong, but complex, genetic component. Genetic investigation of migraine bears great promise in providing new targets for drug development and optimization of individual specific therapy. Better, preferably prophylactic, treatment of migraine patients is desired because the presently used drugs are not effective in all patients, allow recurrence of the headache in a high percentage of patients and sometimes have severe adverse side effects. With the recent identification of the brain-specific P/Q-type calcium channel gene CACNA1A in the pathogenesis of migraine, the first step has been taken to identify primary biochemical pathways leading to migraine. Here, we summarize the current knowledge about the genetics of migraine and focus on the implication for treatment approaches.

Introduction

Migraine is a common paroxysmal disorder, with a one-year prevalence of 6–8% in males and 18–25% in females (Stewart et al., 1992; Launer et al., 1999). Two main, overlapping, sub-types exist: (i) migraine without aura, characterized by unilateral pulsating headache accompanied by either nausea, vomiting and/or photo- and phonophobia; and, (Table 1) migraine with aura, where these symptoms are preceded by visual and/or sensory hallucinations (Headache Classification Committee, 1988; Russell and Olesen, 1996).

Genetic factors are involved in migraine, especially in the aura sub-type, since first-degree relatives of migraineurs are at higher risk of being affected as well (Russell et al., 1995; Haan et al., 1997). Studies with twins also support a genetic component. However, the inheritance pattern is complex, and internal and external environmental factors may trigger symptoms; this defines migraine as a multifactorial disorder.

The identification of specific components contributing to a common multifactorial disease is difficult. An attractive approach is to search for affected genes in a severe, Mendelian-inherited variant of the disorder. A few years ago this was done successfully for migraine by studying families with the rare

Table 1. IHS classification and diagnostic criteria for migraine without aura, migraine with aura and familial hemiplegic migraine

Migraine without aura

A. At least five attacks fulfilling B-D
B. Headache attacks lasting 4–72 hours (untreated or unsuccessfully treated)
C. Headache has at least two of the following characteristics:
   1. Unilateral location
   2. Pulsating quality
   3. Moderate or severe intensity (inhibits or prohibits daily activities)
   4. Aggravation by walking stairs or similar routine physical activity
D. During headache at least one of the following:
   1. Nausea and/or vomiting
   2. Photophobia and phonophobia
E. At least one of the following:
   1. History, physical and neurological examinations do not suggest associated head trauma, vascular or non-vascular intracranial disorders, exposure to or withdrawal from (toxic) substances, non-cephalic infection, metabolic disorders or cranial or facial disorders
   2. History and/or physical- and/or neurological examinations do suggest such disorder, but is ruled out by appropriate investigations
   3. Such disorder is present, but migraine attacks do not occur for the first time in close temporal relation to the disorder

Migraine with aura

A. At least two attacks fulfilling B
B. At least three of the following four characteristics:
   1. One or more fully reversible aura symptoms indicating focal cerebral cortical and/or brain stem dysfunction
   2. At least one aura symptom develops gradually over more than 4 minutes or, two or more symptoms occur in succession
   3. No aura symptom lasts more than 60 minutes. If more than one aura symptom is present, accepted duration is proportionally increased
   4. Headache follows aura with a free interval of less than 60 minutes. (It may also begin before or simultaneously with the aura).
C. At least one of the following:
   1. History, physical and neurological examinations do not suggest associated head trauma, vascular or non-vascular intracranial disorders, exposure to or withdrawal from (toxic) substances, non-cephalic infection, metabolic disorders or cranial or facial disorders
   2. History and/or physical- and/or neurological examinations do suggest such disorder, but is ruled out by appropriate investigations
   3. Such disorder is present, but migraine attacks do not occur for the first time in close temporal relation to the disorder

Familial Hemiplegic migraine

A. Fulfills criteria for migraine with aura
B. The aura includes some degree of hemiparesis and may be prolonged
C. At least one first degree relative has identical attacks

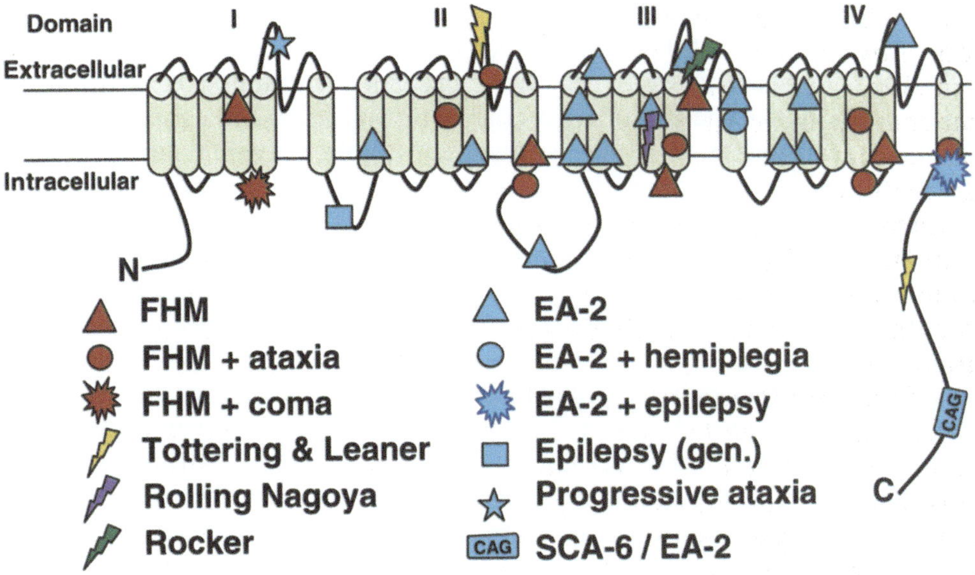

Fig. 1. The CACNA1A clinical spectrum

disorder, familial hemiplegic migraine (FHM) (Ophoff et al., 1996). This disease is autosomal dominantly inherited and has features that are similar to typical migraine with aura, additionally with hemiplegia (one-sided paralysis) during the attacks (Headache Classification Committee, 1988). In about 20% of the FHM families, permanent cerebellar ataxia is present. Initially, FHM was shown to be linked to chromosome 19p13 in about 50% of the families (Joutel et al., 1993; Ophoff et al., 1994). A fraction of FHM families appears to be linked to chromosome 1q and to other loci since in a number of families there is no linkage to either chromosome 19p or 1q (Ducres et al., 1997; Gardner et al., 1997).

In chromosome 19 linked families mutations in the *CACNA1A* gene, coding for α_{1A}, the pore-forming sub-unit of neuronal P/Q-type Ca^{2+} channels were identified (Ophoff et al., 1996). The same study revealed *CACNA1A* mutations in EA-2, a disease characterized by acetazolamide-responsive attacks of cerebellar ataxia. The third autosomal dominant disease in which *CACNA1A* mutations were identified is SCA-6 (Zhuchenko et al., 1997). Clinically, FHM, EA-2 and SCA-6 form a symptomatic spectrum with overlapping, as well as distinct, features.

Many different *CACNA1A* mutations have been identified in families with FHM and EA-2 (Fig. 1). In FHM, these are all missense mutations leading to a single amino acid change in α_{1A} (Ducros et al., 1999, 2001; Terwindt et al., 1998; Elliott et al., 1996). The identified EA2 mutations are predicted to result in the truncation of the α_{1A} protein (Ophoff et al., 1996). In SCA-6, which has considerable clinical overlap with EA-2, mild CAG expansions, 21 to 40 repeats (normally 4 to 17 repeats) have been shown in

CACNA1A, leading to polyglutamine stretches in the intracellular C-terminal domain of the α_{1A} protein (Zhuchenko et al., 1997).

With the identification of an increasing number of mutations in CACNA1A, genotype-phenotype correlation studies have become feasible (Table 2). Terwindt et al. (1998) compared the phenotypical consequences of the FHM I1811L and the V714A mutations. Cerebellar ataxia was observed only with the I1811L mutation (Terwindt et al., 1998). No other significant differences could be identified, except that loss of consciousness during attacks was reported more often in patients with the V714A mutation. Patients with the T666M mutation have been reported with both increased loss of consciousness and cerebellar ataxia (Ducros et al., 1999, 2001). Permanent cerebellar ataxia was also reported in FHM patients with mutations D715E, R583Q, R1668W and W1683R. In contrast, ataxia was never observed with mutations R192Q, V714A, K133E, V1457L and V1695I. Although the number of patients with the mutations mentioned above is very small it seems that the position of the mutation and/or the specific amino acid change controls the development of ataxia in a yet unknown manner.

P/Q-type Ca^{2+} channels and neuropathological α_{1A} mutations

Voltage-dependent Ca^{2+} channels are key protein structures in neuronal cell membranes. They transduce electrical signals into a cellular influx of Ca^{2+}, which acts as a second messenger in many processes such as regulation of excitability, transmitter release, gene regulation and axonal growth. Ca^{2+} channels consist of a pore-forming, voltage-sensing α_1 subunit, and auxiliary β, $\alpha_2\delta$ and γ subunits. Several sub-types of heteromultimeric channels exist, which are discriminated using pharmacological and electrophysiological criteria (ie, N-, P/Q-, L-, R- and T-types). The α_1 subunit consists of four homologous repeats (I to IV), each with six transmembrane segments (S1 to S6, Fig. 1). The so-called P-loop between S5 and S6 is thought to form the inner lining of the ion pore. The S4 segments have been shown to be involved in voltage sensing (Bezanilla, 2000).

The *CACNA1A* gene encodes for the pore-forming subunit, α_{1A}. Alternative splicing of *CACNA1A* yields either P- or Q-type channels (Bourinet et al., 1999). P/Q-type Ca^{2+} channels are widely expressed in the central nervous system, especially in the cerebellum (Westenbroek et al., 1995). In cell bodies, P/Q-type Ca^{2+} channels play a role in excitability, presumably via Ca^{2+}-dependent K^+ channels. Furthermore, Ca^{2+} influx stimulates intracellular signaling pathways, mostly involving kinases, which can influence gene expression, for example (Bito, 1998). During development, P/Q-type Ca^{2+} channels seem to participate in the process of neurite initiation (Heng et al., 1999). At mature synaptic terminals, their main function is to mediate transmitter secretion by allowing Ca^{2+} to stimulate the release-machinery complex at so-called active zones, resulting in exocytosis of synaptic vesicles (Sudhof, 1995). The α_{1A} subunit contains defined sites that interact with specific presynaptic proteins (Fig. 1), presumably required for targeted presynaptic localization and specific presynaptic function of P/Q-type Ca^{2+} channels (Catterall, 1999; Lee et al., 1999; Maximov et al., 1999).

P/Q-type Ca^{2+}-channel mutant mice

A number of mice models exist with natural or induced mutations in *Cacnala* (Fig. 1). These are the *tottering* (missense P601L) *leaner* (splice-site mutation, leading to aberrant and shortened cytoplasmatic C-terminal), *rolling Nagoya* (missense R1262G), *rocker* (missense T1310K) and null-mutant mice (Doyle et al., 1997; Fletcher et al., 1996; Mori et al., 2000; Zwingmann et al., 2001; Fletcher et al., 2001; Jun et al., 1999). They all display ataxia and, except for *rolling Nagoya*, signs of epilepsy. *Leaner*, *rolling Nagoya* and null-mutant mice develop cerebellar degeneration. *Leaner* and null-mutant mice die at about 3 weeks of age. As yet, the *Cacnala*-mutant mice seem to be the best available models for FHM and related diseases and several studies have been performed to analyze the behavior of their P/Q-type Ca^{2+} channels.

Functional consequences of mutations in CACNA1A

The genetic findings in migraine in mice and men have strongly directed the migraine field towards studying the functional consequences of mutant P/Q-type Ca^{2+} channels, aiming to unravel genotype-phenotype relations and to gain insight into the role of P/Q-type Ca^{2+} channels in pathophysiological mechanisms of migraine. It is also very likely that it is possible to use the newly acquired knowledge to develop new migraine therapies.

So far, the functional consequences of only a few mutations in the CACNA1A gene have been studied. Abnormalities in calcium channel function can be investigated by measuring disturbances in electrophysiological parameters using patch clamp techniques, either on the whole-cell level or by single channel measurements. Mutations have been introduced in either the rabbit or human cDNA and were transfected in *Xenopus* oocytes or human embryonic kidney 293 cells. Different mutations in CACNA1A cause an identical clinical phenotype, suggesting that these mutations might have a similar effect on calcium channel functioning: a loss-of-function or gain-of-function. However, results from two research groups have shown very complicated patterns for the individual mutants (Kraus et al., 1998, 2000; Hans et al., 1999) (Table 3).

Certain parameters, such as the voltage at which the mutant channels open, did change in the same direction for most of the mutations tested. Mutated Ca^{2+} channels are opened already at weak depolarisations. However, other parameters, like channel inactivation or the recovery from inactivation, showed different effects for the various mutations. In addition, the expression level of functionally active channels varied considerably among the mutations.

Mutation R192Q results in a 2-fold increase in current, that is mainly due to an increased expression of mutated channels on the plasma membrane and

Table 2. FHM mutations in the CACNA1A gene and clinical phenotypic variation

Amino acid	Exon	Localisation	Ataxia	Additional notes
R192Q	4	IS4	−	
R583Q	13	IIS4	+	Second frequent mutation; No common haplotype in four families → altered consciousness → Acetazolamide-responsive
T666M	16	IIS5–S6 linker	+	Most frequent mutation; No common haplotype in over 10 families Also sporadic case observed → interictal nystagmus
V714A	17	IIS6	−	
D715E	17	Loop II–III	+	→ Essential tremor
*K1335E	25	IIIS3–S4 linker	−	
*Y1384C	26	IIIS5	+	Sporadic case Partial seizures, meningism, fever, altered consciousness; Moderate mental deficit, nystagmus
V1457L	27	IIIS5–S6 linker	−	
*R1667W	32	IVS4	−	
*L1682P	32	IVS4–S5 linker	+	→ Interictal nystagmus
*W1683R	32	IVS4–S5 linker	+	
V1695I	33	IVS5	−	
I1811L	36	IVS6	+	

Specific amino acid substitutions are indicated; *: publication in abstract form with only partial clinical information; amino acid positions are given according to Genbank Accession Number X99897. Ataxia +: ataxia is an additional prominent symptom observed in these FHM patients; ataxia −: ataxia is not observed in these FHM patients. Additional notes: → phenotypic variation observed with some of the carriers of the mutation

Table 3. Functional consequences of FHM mutations

Mutation	Activation voltage	Steady-state Inactivation kinetics	Inactivation time constant	Channel inactivation during pulse trains	Recovery from inactivation time constant	Peak current density	Channel density on plasma membrane*	Most likely consequence of mutation on calcium influx
R192Q	↔	↔	↔	↔	↔	↑	↑	Gain-of-function
R583Q	Negative Shift	Negative Shift	↔	↑	↑	↓	Not determined	Loss-of-function
T666M	Negative Shift	↔	↑	↑	↑	↓	↓	Loss-of-function
V714A	Negative Shift	↔	↑	↓	↓	↓	↓	Gain or-Loss-of-function
D715E	Negative Shift	Negative Shift	↑	↑	↔	↓	Not determined	Loss-of-function
V1457L	Negative Shift	↔	↓	↔	↑	↓	Not determined	Gain or-Loss-of-function
I1811L	Negative Shift	↔	↔	↓	↓	↓	↓	Gain or-Loss-of-function

The changes are in respect to wildtype calcium channels. In all cases, ↔: not different from wildtype; ↓: less than wildtype; ↑: more than wildtype. * All data are from Kraus et al. (1998, 2000), except for channel density on the membrane (Hans et al., 1999)

to a lesser extent to an increased open probability of the channels at all voltages. So, it is expected that more calcium ions enter through such a mutated channel.

In contrast, the T666M mutation shows both a strongly decreased expression of functionally active channels, as well as a reduced single-channel current. This explains the observed reduced whole-cell current density. As a result, calcium influx is probably lower with this mutation than in the wildtype situation. More difficult to understand are the functional consequences of the V714A and I1811L mutations. The V714A mutation and, to a lesser extent, the I1811L mutation allow channel opening at more negative potentials combined with an increased open probability. This would imply that more calcium ions enter the cell through a single channel. However, when these data are combined with the reduced expression of channels with these mutations (~40% and ~20% of wildtype expression, respectively), it remains unclear whether this increased single-channel influx is counterbalanced at the whole cell level by reduced channel expression.

The question arises if any of the altered biophysical properties could account for the episodic character of migraine. Indeed, for mutations R583Q, T666M, V714A, D715E, and I1811L an increased or decreased Ca^{2+} current decay was observed during rapid trains of depolarizations. This was changed to altered channel inactivation during individual test pulses and/or changes in the recovery from inactivated channel states between pulses. It is therefore likely that pronounced alterations in neuronal Ca^{2+} influx occur in FHM neurons especially during episodes of high neuronal activity. This mechanism could link excessive neuronal stimulation (e.g. induced by migraine triggers) to the neuronal instability observed in functional studies.

It is difficult to predict the amount of calcium ions that enter a specific neuronal cell containing mutated P/Q-type calcium channels. Many additional parameters, such as 1) the relative expression of the mutant and wildtype channel protein in a given neuronal cell, 2) the contribution of various splice forms of the CACNA1A calcium channel subunit, 3) the contribution of (alternatively spliced) auxillary subunits, have not been studied yet.

Also the strange observation that some mutated channels can switch modes as function of time and seem to function as wildtype channels during short time periods, is not well understood and might be of importance (Hans et al., 1999). At present, we do not know whether compensatory mechanisms are operational, when these mutated calcium channels are expressed in neuronal nerve terminals or soma together with other channels like L-type and N-type calcium channels.

Implications for insight in migraine pathophysiology

One of the major questions is how mutated calcium channels cause FHM and are related to the common forms of migraine. From electrophysiological studies described above, one might suggest that disturbances in calcium channels result in either an increase or a decrease of calcium ion flux into neuronal cells. These abnormalities in calcium channel functioning could result in neuronal instability which renders patients susceptible to migraine attacks, triggered by external factors. The observation that the functional disturbances were more prominent at high frequency stimulation, gives an explanation as to the episodic nature of the associated disease. In FHM patients with V714A or I1811L mutations, sustained neuronal firing due to an incorrect integration of (otherwise normal) neural stimuli might result in a relative decreased inactivation of calcium channels. Ultimately, this will result in an increased influx of calcium ions and perhaps abnormal down stream neuronal signalling pathways. Abnormal Ca2+ influx can very well explain the observed cell death resulting in cerebellar atrophy.

As P/Q-type calcium channels control neurotransmitter release from nerve terminals (including serotoninergic caudal raphe neurons, it will be important to prove that altered Ca^{2+} influx of FHM mutations translates into changes in neurotransmitter release (Bayliss et al., 1997). This hypothesis is strongly supported by recent findings in *tottering* mice. These mice have a missense mutation changing a Proline into a Leucine at position 601 of the same P/Q-type calcium and are considered models for absence epilepsy (Fletcher et al., 1996). Spontaneous acetylcholine release in peripheral synapses of the neuromuscular junction is increased in *tottering* mice (Plomp et al., 2000). However, at high frequency stimulation, there is a decrease in transmitter release in the homozyous mice. Field-potential studies in thalamic nuclei, and hippocampal areas, show that neurotransmitter release is also altered in the CNS of *tottering* mice (Caddick et al., 1999; Qian and Noebels, 2000). In thalamic nuclei, transmitter release at specifically glutamatergic synapses seem to be reduced (Caddick et al., 1999). Interestingly, a reduced calcium influx through P/Q-type channels, and a coinciding decrease in neurotransmitter release from these channels, does not prevent compensation of neurotransmitter release via N-type channels in *tottering* (Qian and Noebels, 2000). Future studies will have to test whether only neurons that are unable to rely on compensatory mechanisms are compromised in this mouse model.

Although tentative at present, the observation by Ferrari et al. (1989; 1990) that serotonin and glutamate levels in migraine patients are altered, especially during attacks, seems to fit into an integrated hypothesis on migraine pathophysiology that now includes abnormalities in neurotransmitter release due to P/Q-type calcium channel mutations (Ferrari et al., 1989, 1990).

Other genes

A number of association studies in migraine have been published, many of them with conflicting results (Montagna, 2000) Most consistent, however, is the association between migraine and the dopamine D2 receptor (DRD2). Clinical and pharmacological evidence supports the hypothesis that dopamine could be involved in the pathogenesis of migraine (Peroutka, 1997). In a case-control study, association between the DRD2 NcoI C allele and migraine with aura was observed, but not in migraine without aura (Peroutka et al., 1997). This finding failed to be replicated in a small uncontrolled association study published by Dichgans et al. (1998). In a family-based association study in the population isolate of Sardinia, evidence was found, using transmission disequilibrium test (TDT), that the allelic distribution of DRD2 differed significantly in a subgroup of "dopaminergic" patients with migraine without aura suggesting that hypersensitivity of the dopaminergic system could be involved in at least a subgroup of patients (Del Zompo et al., 1998). Dopaminergic migraine patients were selected upon the presence of both nausea and yawning immediately before or during the pain phase of migraine. The fact that two independent studies have shown an association between molecular variations within the DRD2 gene and migraine suggests that genetic variation within dopaminergic system function may underlie clinical susceptibility to migraine. It is clear, however, that additional genetic, biochemical and clinical studies are needed to assess the (putative) role of dopamine in the pathophysiology of migraine. Likewise, contradictory results were found in genetic studies of the serotonergic system.

There are several hereditary diseases in which migraine is a prominent symptom: epilepsy, cluster headache, a new syndrome characterized by autosomal dominant vascular retinopathy, Raynaud's phenomenon and migraine, familial migraine with vertigo and essential tremor, dyslipoproteinemias, hereditary hemorrhagic telangiectasia, Tourette's syndrome, alternating hemiplegia of childhood, several psychiatric disorders, the Stormorken syndrome, hereditary essential tremor, cerebral cavernous malformations, hereditary cerebral amyloid angiopathy, CADASIL, and several movement disorders (Haan et al., 1997). Further study of these diseases might give new clues for the genetic cause of migraine, but no evidence to a contribution to MO or MA of the genes involved in these disorders is present at this moment.

Implications for the treatment of migraine

Different treatment strategies, based on empirical grounds, are currently used to treat migraine attacks (Ferrari, 1998; Diener et al., 1998). Here, the clinical treatment of migraine attacks will be summarized.

Prophylactic treatment of migraine

The most import indications to start prophylaxis are headache frequency of more than 2 attacks per month, no or inappropriate response to acute treatment or when optimal abortive therapies have produced intolerable side effects. Some drugs have been shown effective like, valproic acid and some of the beta-blockers (like propanolol), but the efficacy is limited: at most 55% of patients will have 50% or more reduction of the attack. Other drugs, e.g. calcium channel blockers (e.g. flunarizine) or 5-HT_2 receptor antagonists (e.g. methysergide), seem to be effective, but efficacy has not been evaluated in randomised trials with current methodology (Silberstein, 1998; Toda and Tfelt-Hansen, 2000). Unfortunenately, these drugs show severe side-effects. Clearly, there is a great necessity for better prophylactic agents and well-designed trials are needed to guide the use of these drugs. At present, the mode of action in prophylactic treatment is mostly unknown (Goadsby, 1997).

Acute treatment of migraine

Mild to moderate migraine attacks may be treated by non-specific drugs such as analgesic and rapidly absorbable NSAIDs (Ferrari, 1998; Diener et al., 1998). Especially, the combination of a NSAID such as aspirin and an anti-emetic compound, like metoclopramide, that helps absorption of the drug, has proven highly effective in the treatment of migraine (Tfelt-Hansen et al., 1995). Aspirin and paracetamol are the most frequent used drugs for the treatment of migraine, and combined with caffeine proven to be effective in the treatment of migraine pain and associated symptoms in several placebo-controlled trials (Lipton et al., 1998; Goldstein et al., 1999). The choice of drug, dose, and route of administration, depends on the characteristics and frequency of the attacks, and on the specific preferences and contra-indications of the patient (Ferrari, 1998).

For decades, the only specific drugs for the acute treatment of migraine were ergot alkaloids (e.g. ergotamine). Ergotamine is effective because of its potent vasoconstrictor activity. Although these ergot alkaloids are widely used, their efficacy has been poorly demonstrated by placebo-controlled clinical trials. Still, ergotamine may be useful in certain patients, such as those with prolonged attacks (>48 hours) or in whom headache recurrence is a substantial issue. Use of ergotamines may induce many side effects such as nausea, vomiting, vertigo, gastric symptoms, dry mouth and restlessness. The drug ergotamine has frequently been associated with substernal chest pain, discomfort and even myocardial infarction and sudden death. In addition, overdose or chronic overuse of ergotamine may induce ergotism: cyanosis, necrosis and infarctions of the heart and brain (Meyler, 1996). A more frequent side effect is ergot-dependent headache that can be induced even by small doses of ergots, if taken regularly twice or more times a week (Meyler, 1996). The high occurrence of side effects is probably due to the wide range of receptors (e.g. α-adrenoreceptor, dopamine and serotonin receptors) to which ergots display affinity (Meyler, 1996). More detailed characterization of the ergotamine receptor pathways may provide clues to response improvement in individual cases (e.g. receptor polymorphisms) and the development of more specific derivative structures to achieve better specificity and efficacy. Ergot alkaloids have low oral and rectal bioavailability and clinical response is not related to plasma concentration of the drug (Tfelt-Hansen et al., 1985).

Sumatriptan is the first migraine drug for which a specific molecular basis of action is known (Humphrey et al., 1990). It was designed to act selectively as a vasoconstrictor at 5-HT1 receptors in cranial blood vessels, but the drug also acts on 5-HT1 receptors located in peripheral human blood vessels. The exact mode of action of sumatriptan, however, is still under debate. Three distinct modes of action have been suggested:

- Vasoconstriction of meningeal, dural, cerebral, or pial vessels, mediated via stimulation of vascular 5-HT_{1B} receptors.
- Inhibition of dural neurogenic inflammation, most probably mediated by presynaptic stimulation of 5-HT_{1D} and/or 5-HT_{1F} receptors.
- Central inhibition of pain transmission: inhibition of trigeminal neurons in the brain stem and upper spinal cord, mediated by 5-HT_{1B}, 5-HT_{1D} or 5-HT_{1F} receptors.

The discovery of sumatriptan was a major improvement in acute treatment of migraine. The drug is highly effective and well-tolerated (Ferrari, 1991). However, sumatriptan has some shortcomings such as low oral bioavailability and recurrence of headache within 24 to 48 hours after initial headache relief in up to 40% of patients with initial good response (Ferrari and Saxena, 1993, 1995). Still, up to 15% of patients never respond to subcutaneous sumatriptan. Importantly, up to about 40% of patients report chest-related symptoms, when specially asked for it (Visser et al., 1996). Other adverse events that have frequently been reported are e.g. tingling, paraesthesias, and warm sensations in the head, neck, chest and limbs. In exceptional cases, more severe side effects have been reported such as myocardial infarction and cardiac arrest. This is the main reason why the drug is contra-indicated in patients with coronary artery disease because of its potential to constrict coronary arteries (MaassenVanDenBrink et al., 1999). Based on success of sumatriptan, second-generation triptans have been developed with similar pharmacodynamic characteristics. The main differences between these compounds are determined by their different pharmacokinetics. Compared to sumatriptan, the oral bioavailability is much higher (45–75%) and thus more consistent and the therapeutic plasma levels are reached more rapidly (30–60 minutes). In addition, the second generation triptans show increased lipophilicity and brain penetration. However, the main characteristic of all available triptans for the acute treatment remains the ability to contract blood vessels and to prevent secondary symptoms.

The development of new generation triptans with improved characteristics and specificity can be guided by the rapidly increasing knowledge on the heterogeneity and function of the 5HT receptor superfamily (Dichgans et al., 1998). Equally, identification of functional polymorphisms in these receptors may help to explain inter-individual differences in response and side effects. First, relevant published data on the use pharmacogenetics in migraine was reported by MaassenVanDenBrink et al. (1998) who studied the possible relation between 5-HT_{1B} polymorphisms (G861C and T-261G) and the clinical response to sumatriptan in various groups of migraine patients, but did not observe a significant difference (MaassenVanDenBrink et al., 1998). Interestingly, two polymorphisms in serotonin receptor 5-HT-1B (F124C) and 5-HT-2C (C23S) have been shown to negatively affect for instance binding of dihydroergotamine, sumatriptan and serotonin, respectively and therefore might be good starting points for future pharmacogenetic studies in migraine patients (Brüss et al., 1999; Lappalainen et al., 1995). As a consequence of the above mentioned genetic discoveries in migraine, also ion channels are good candidates to be studied as new drug target. Thus far, no specific treatment has resulted from these studies, but the aspecific carbonanhydrase inhibitor acetazolamide seems to have some effect in migraine.

Future studies

To complete the molecular portrait of migraine pathogenesis, additional genes have to be identified and their function determined. It is likely that the next several years will surface novel candidate genes. Already, a novel FHM locus has been identified on chromosomes 1q. It is of course only speculation what the next migraine gene might look like. Likely candidates are calcium channel subunits, genes implicated in calcium metabolism or neurotransmitter release mechanisms, thereby reinforcing the concept that migraine is a channelopathy. Of course, such a gene can also have a completely different role, revealing a completely new insight into migraine pathophysiology. Complementary strategies to identify such genes are being followed in our and other laboratories. The most straightforward approach is to map genes by parametric linkage analysis in families with a Mendelian inheritance pattern as demonstrated by our work in FHM. This approach has also been applied to map migraine with aura genes. However, considering the high prevalence of migraine, the clinical heterogeneity of migraine and available population-based estimates of heritability based on segregation and twin studies, more large-scale non-parametric linkage and association methods have to be applied. The rapid progress of the Human Genome Project with dense genetic marker high-throughput genotyping technology, the use of common DNA variations named single-nucleotide polymorphisms (SNPs) in combination with advanced biostatistical methods will crucially facilitate such approaches (McCarthy and Hilfiker, 2000). In spite of the unprecedented capacity from the laboratory side, the success will however be instrumentally dependent on the quality of well-characterized patient material; families as well as patient cohorts. The coming decades will show whether these pharmacogenetic approaches have yielded more specific and efficous treatment of migraine patients with less side effects.

References

Bayliss DA, Li YW, Talley EM (1997) Effects of serotonin on caudal raphe neurons: inhibition of N- and P/Q-type calcium channels and the after hyperpolarization. J Neurophysiol 77: 1362–1374

Bezanilla F (2000) The voltage sensor in voltage-dependent ion channels. Physiol Rev 80: 555–592

Bito H (1998) The role of calcium in activity-dependent neuronal gene regulation. Cell Calcium 23: 143–150

Bourinet E, Soong TW, Sutton K, Slaymaker S, Mathews E, Monteil A, Zamponi GW, Nargeot J, Snutch TP (1999) Splicing of alpha 1A subunit gene generates phenotypic variants of P- and Q-type calcium channels. Nature Neurosci 2: 407–415

Brüss M, Bönisch H, Bühlen, Nöthen MM, Propping P, Göthert M (1999) Modified ligand binding to the naturally occurring Cys 124 variant of the human serotonin 5-HT_{1B} receptor. Pharmacogenetics 9: 95–102

Caddick SJ, Wang C, Fletcher CF, Jenkins NA, Copeland NG, Hosford DA (1999) Excitatory but not inhibitory synaptic transmission is reduced in lethargic (Cacnb4(lh)) and tottering (Cacnalatg) mouse thalami. J Neurophysiol 81: 2066–2074

Catterall WA (1999) Interactions of presynaptic Ca^{2+} channels and snare proteins in neurotransmitter release. Ann NY Acad Sci 868: 144–159

Del Zompo M, Cherchi A, Palmas MA, Ponti M, Bocchetta A, Gessa GL, Piccardi MP (1998) Association between dopamine receptor genes and migraine without aura in a Sardinian sample. Neurology 51: 781–786

Dichgans M, Forderreuther S, Deiterich M, Pfaffenrath V, Gasser T (1998) The D2 receptor NcoI allele: absence of allelic association with migraine with aura. Neurology 51: 928

Diener HC, Kaube H, Limmroth V (1998) A practical guide to the management and prevention of migraine. Drugs 56: 811–824

Doyle J, Ren X, Lennon G, Stubbs L (1997) Mutations in the Cacnl1a4 calcium channel gene are associated with seizures, cerebellar degeneration, and ataxia in tottering and leaner mutant mice. Mamm Genome 8: 113–120

Ducros A, Joutel A, Vahedi K, Cecillon M, Ferreira A, Bernard E, Verier A, Echenne B, Lopez de Munain A, Bousser MG, Tournier-Lasserve E (1997) Mapping of a second locus for familial hemiplegic migraine to 1q21–q23 and evidence of further heterogeneity. Ann Neurol 42: 885–890

Ducros A, Denier C, Joutel A, Vahedi K, Bousser M-G, Tournier-Lasserve E (1999) Characterization of CACNA1A mutations in familial and sporadic hemiplegic migraine. Neurology 52 [Suppl 2]: A273–274

Ducros A, Denier C, Joutel A, Vahedi K, Michel A, Darcel F, Madigand M, Guerouaou D, Tison F, Julien J, Hirsch E, Chedru F, Bisgard C, Lucotte G, Despres P, Billard C, Barthez MA, Ponsot G, Bousser MG, Tournier-Lasserve E (1999) Recurrence of the T666M calcium channel CACNA1A gene mutation in familial hemiplegic migraine with progressive cerebellar ataxia. Am J Hum Genet 64: 89–98

Ducros A, Denier C, Joutel A, et al. (2001) The clinical spectrum of familial hemiplegic migraine associated with mutations in a neuronal calcium channel. N Engl J Med 345: 17–24

Elliott MA, Peroutka SJ, Welch S, May EF (1996) Familial hemiplegic migraine, nystagmus, and cerebellar atrophy Ann Neurol 39: 100–106

Ferrari MD (1998) Migraine. Lancet 351: 1043–1051

Ferrari MD, for the Subcutaneous Sumatriptan International Study Group (1991) Treatment of migraine attacks with sumatriptan. N Engl J Med 325: 316–321

Ferrari MD, Saxena PR (1993) Clinical and experimental effects of sumatriptan in humans. Trends Pharmacol Sci 14: 129–133

Ferrari MD, Saxena PR (1995) 5-HT1 receptors in migraine pathophysiology and treatment. Eur J Neurol 2: 5–21

Ferrari MD, Odink J, Tapparelli C, Van Kempen GM, Pennings EJ, Bruyn GW (1989) Serotonin metabolism in migraine. Neurology 39: 1239–1242

Ferrari MD, Odink J, Bos KD, Malessy MJ, Bruyn GW (1990) Neuroexcitatory plasma amino acids are elevated in migraine. Neurology 40: 1582–1586

Fletcher CF, Lutz CM, O'Sullivan TN, Shaughnessy JD, Hawkes R, Frankel WN, Copeland NG, Jenkins NA (1996) Absence epilepsy in tottering mutant mice is associated with calcium channel defects. Cell 87: 607–617

Fletcher CF, Tottene A, Lennon VA, Wilson SM, Dubel SJ, Paylor R, Hosford DA, Tessarollo L, McEnery MW, Pietrobon D, Copeland NG, Jenkins NA (2001) Dystonia and cerebellar atrophy in Cacna1a null mice lacking P/Q calcium channel activity. FASEB J 15: 1288–1290

Gardner K, Barmada MM, Ptacek LJ, Hoffman EP (1997) A new locus for hemiplegic migraine maps to chromosome 1q31. Neurology 49: 1231–1238

Goadsby PJ (1997) How do the currently used prophylactic agents work in migraine? Cephalalgia 17: 85–92

Goldstein J, Hoffman HD, Armellino JJ, Battikha JP, Hamelsky SW, Couch J, Blumenthal H, Lipton RB (1999) Treatment of severe, disabling migraine attacks in over-the-counter population of migraine sufferers: results from three randomized, placebo-controlled studies of the combination of acetaminophen, aspirin, and caffeine. Cephalalgia 19: 684–691

Haan J, Terwindt GM, Ferrari MD (1997) Genetics of migraine. In: Mathew NT (ed) Neurological clinics. Saunders, Philadelphia, pp 43–60 (Adv Headache)

Hans M, Luvisetto S, Williams ME, Spagnolo M, Urrutia A, Tottene A, Brust PF, Johnson EC, Harpold MM, Stauderman KA, Pietrobon D (1999) Functional consequences of mutations in the human α1A calcium channel subunit linked to familial hemiplegic migraine. J Neurosci 9: 1610–1619

Headache Classification Committee of the International Headache Society (1988) Classification and diagnostic criteria for headache disorders, cranial neuralgias and facial pain. Cephalalgia 8: 1–97

Heng JE, Zurakowski D, Vorwerk CK, Grosskreutz CL, Dreyer EB (1999) Cation channel control of neurite morphology. Dev Brain Res 113: 67–73

Humphrey PP, Feniuk W, Perren MJ, Beresford IJ, Skingle M, Whalley ET (1990) Serotonin and migraine. Ann NY Acad Sci 600: 587–600

Joutel A, Bousser MG, Biousse V, Labauge P, Chabriat H, Nibbio A, Maciazek J, Meyer B, Bach MA, Weissenbach J, Latrop GM, Tournier-Lasserve E (1993) A gene for familial hemiplegic migraine maps to chromosome 19. Nat Genet 5: 40–45

Jun K, Piedras-Renteria ES, Smith SM, Wheeler DB, Lee SB, Lee TG, Chin H, Adams ME, Scheller RH, Tsien RW, Shin HS (1999) Ablation of P/Q-type Ca(2+) channel currents, altered synaptic transmission, and progressive ataxia in mice lacking the alpha(1A)-subunit. Proc Natl Acad Sci USA 96: 15245–15250

Kraus RL, Sinnegger MJ, Glossmann H, Hering S, Striessnig J (1998) Familial hemiplegic migraine mutations change α1A Ca^{2+} channel kinetics. J Biol Chem 273: 5586–5590

Kraus RL, Sinnegger MJ, Koschak A, Glossmann H, Stenirri S, Carrera P, Striessnig J (2000) Three new familial hemiplegic migraine mutants affect P/Q-type Ca(2+) channel kinetics. J Biol Chem 275: 9239–9243

Lappalainen J, Zhang L, Dean M, Oz M, Ozaki N, Yu D-H, Virkkunen M, Weight F, Linnoila M, Goldman D (1995) Identification, expression, and pharmacology of a Cys23-Ser23 substitution in the human 5-HT_{2C} receptor gene (HTR_{2C}). Genomics 2: 274–279

Launer LJ, Terwindt GM, Ferrari MD (1999) The prevalence and characteristics of migraine in a population based cohort: the GEM study. Neurology 53: 537–542

Lee A, Wong ST, Gallagher D, Li B, Storm DR, Scheuer T, Catterall WA (1999) Ca^{2+}/calmodulin binds to and modulates P/Q-type calcium channels. Nature 399: 155–159

Lipton RB, Stewart WF, Ryan RE Jr, Saper J, Silberstein S, Sheftell F (1998) Efficacy and safety of randomized, placebo-controlled trials. Arch Neurol 55: 210–217

MaassenVanDenBrink A, Vergouwe MN, Ophoff RA, Saxena PR, Ferrari MD, Frants RR (1998) 5-HT_{1B} receptor polymorphisms and clinical response to sumatriptan. Headache 38: 288–291

MaassenVanDenBrink A, Bax WA, Ramrattan NN, Ferrari MD, Saxena PR (1999) Human coronary artery contraction to sumatriptan: a post hoc analysis. Cephalalgia 9: 651–654

Maximov A, Sudhof TC, Bezprozvanny I (1999) Association of neuronal calcium channels with modular adaptor proteins. J Biol Chem 274: 24453–24456
McCarthy JJ, Hilfiker R (2000) The use of single-nucleotide polymorphism maps in harmacogenomics. Nature Biotech 8: 505–508
Meyler WJ (1996) Side effects of ergotamine. Cephalalgia 16: 5–10
Montagna P (2000) Molecular genetics of migraine headaches: a review. Cephalalgia 20: 3–14
Mori Y, Wakamori M, Oda S, Fletcher CF, Sekiguchi N, Mori E, Copeland NG, Jenkins NA, Matsushita K, Matsuyama Z, Imoto K (2000) Reduced voltage sensitivity of activation of P/Q-type Ca^{2+} channels is associated with the ataxic mouse mutation rolling Nagoya (tg(rol)). J Neurosci 20: 5654–5662
Ophoff RA, van Eijk R, Sandkuijl LA, Terwindt GM, Grubben CP, Haan J, Lindhout D, Ferrari MD, Frants RR (1994) Genetic heterogeneity of familial hemiplegic migraine. Genomics 22: 21–26
Ophoff RA, Terwindt GM, Vergouwe MN, van Eijk R, Oefner PJ, Hoffman SM, Lamerdin JE, Mohrenweiser HW, Bulman DE, Ferrari M, Haan J, Lindhout D, van Ommen GJ, Hofker MH, Ferrari MD, Frants RR (1996) Familial hemiplegic migraine and episodic ataxia type-2 are caused by mutations in the Ca^{2+} channel gene CACNL1A4. Cell 87: 543–552
Peroutka SJ (1997) Dopamine and migraine. Neurology 49: 650–656
Peroutka SJ, Wilhoit T, Jones K (1997) Clinical susceptibility to migraine with aura is modified by dopamine D2 receptor (DRD2) NcoI alleles. Neurology 49: 201–206
Plomp JJ, Vergouwe MN, Van den Maagdenberg AM, Ferrari MD, Frants RR, Molenaar PC (2000) Abnormal transmitter release at neuromuscular junctions of mice carrying the tottering α(1A) Ca(2+) channel mutation. Brain 123(Pt 3): 463–471
Qian J, Noebels JL (2000) Presynaptic Ca(2+) influx at a mouse central synapse with Ca(2+) channel subunit mutations. J Neurosci 20: 163–170
Russell MB, Olesen J (1996) A nosographic analysis of the migraine aura in a general population. Brain 119: 355–361
Russell MB, Iselius L, Olesen J (1995) Inheritance of migraine investigated by complex segregation analysis. Hum Genet 96: 726–730
Silberstein SD (1998) Methysergide. Cephalalgia 8: 421–435
Stewart WF, Lipton RB, Celentano DD, Reed ML (1992) Prevalence of migraine headache in the United States: relation to age, income, race and other sociodemographic factors. J Am Med Assoc 267: 64–69
Sudhof TC (1995) The synaptic vesicle cycle: a cascade of protein-protein interactions. Nature 375: 645–653
Terwindt GM, Ophoff RA, Haan J, Vergouwe MN, van Eijk R, Frants RR, Ferrari MD (1998) Variable clinical expression of mutations in the P/Q-type calcium channel gene in familial hemiplegic migraine. Dutch Migraine Genetics Research Group. Neurology 50: 1105–1110
Tfelt-Hansen P, Paalzow L (1985) Intramuscular ergotamine: plasma levels and dynamic activity. Clin Pharmacol Ther 37: 29–35
Tfelt-Hansen P, Henry P, Mulder LJ, Scheldewaert RG, Schoenen J, Chazot G (1995) The effectiveness of combined oral lysine acetylsalicylate and metoclopramide compared with oral sumatriptan for migraine. Lancet 346: 923–926
Toda N, Tfelt-Hansen P (2000) Calcium antagonists in migraine prophylaxis. In: Olesen J, Tfelt-Hansen P, Welch KMA (eds) The headaches, 2nd edn. Lippincott Williams & Wilkins, Philadelphia, pp 477–487
Visser WH, Jaspers NMWH, Vriend de RHM, Ferrari MD (1996) Chest symptoms after sumatriptan: a two-years clinical practice review in 735 consecutive migraine patients. Cephalalgia 16: 554–559
Westenbroek RE, Sakurai T, Elliott EM, Hell JW, Starr TV, Snutch TP, Catterall WA (1995) Immunochemical identification and subcellular distribution of the alpha 1A subunits of brain calcium channels. J Neurosci 15: 6403–6418

Zhuchenko O, Bailey J, Bonnen P, Ashizawa T, Stockton DW, Amos C, Dobyns WB, Subramony SH, Zoghbi HY, Lee CC (1997) Autosomal dominant cerebellar ataxia (SCA6) associated with small polyglutamine expansions in the alpha 1A-voltage-dependent calcium channel. Nat Genet 15: 62–69

Zwingman TA, Neumann PE, Noebels JL, Herrup K (2001) Rocker is a new variant of the voltage-dependent calcium channel gene Cacna1a. J Neurosci 21: 1169–1178

Authors' address: M.D. Ferrari, MD PhD, Department of Neurology, K-5-Q, Leiden University Medical Center, PO Box 9600, 2300 RC Leiden, The Netherlands, e-mail: M.D.Ferrari@lumc.nl

J Neural Transm (2002) [Suppl] 63: 129–147

Does schizophrenia result from developmental or degenerative processes?

S. M. Church, D. Cotter, E. Bramon, and **R. M. Murray**

Institute of Psychiatry, De Crespigny Park, London, United Kingdom

Summary. The debate as to whether schizophrenia is a neurodevelopmental or a neurodegenerative disorder has its roots in the latter part of the 19th century when authorities such as Clouston (1891) posited that at least some insanities were "developmental" in origin. These views were soon eclipsed by Kraepelin's (1896) concept of dementia praecox as a degenerative disease, and the latter view carried not only the day but also much of the 20th century. Then, in the 1980s several research groups again began to speculate that schizophrenia might have a significant developmental component (Feinberg, 1982–1983; Schulsinger et al., 1984; Murray et al., 1985; Murray and Lewis, 1987; Weinberger et al., 1987). What became known as the "neurodevelopmental hypothesis" received support from neuropathological studies implicating anomalies in early brain development such as aberrant migration of neurons. Unfortunately, these studies proved difficult, if not impossible, to replicate (Harrison, 1999).

The pendulum, therefore, began to swing again, and in the latter part of the 1990s came renewed claims that the clinical progression of the illness was accompanied by continued cerebral ventricular enlargement and reduction in the volumes of certain brain structures. Nevertheless, since few doubt that there is a developmental component to schizophrenia, the question which we will address in this paper is whether schizophrenia is a) simply the final consequence of a cascade of increasing developmental deviance (Bramon et al., 2001), or b) whether there is an additional brain degeneration following onset of psychosis which is superimposed on the developmental impairment (Lieberman, 1999).

The case for impaired neurodevelopment

When the term "neurodevelopmental" is applied to schizophrenia, it can be used with two different meanings. Firstly, in a static temporal sense to refer to a process damaging the brain at a specific time and leaving a static deficit. The abnormality is thought to occur either during foetal or neonatal life (early developmental theory), or during adolescent brain maturation (late developmental theory). Both versions assume that, following onset, the illness runs its course with no further neurobiological consequences other than those of normal maturation, ageing, and the effects of treatment.

The second meaning of the term neurodevelopmental is that of an abnormal neural process continuing throughout childhood and adolescence which results ultimately in the onset of psychosis (Woods, 1998). Since this process may or may not stop at the onset of psychotic symptoms, this meaning of the term is compatible with an ongoing pathological process continuing during the disease.

Early developmental theories

The developmental theories proposed in the mid-1980s, postulated that aetiological factors operate early in life, long before the onset of psychosis. These factors disrupt the course of neural development, leading to alterations of specific neurones and the circuits they form (Weinberger, 1987; Murray and Lewis, 1987), and a "neurodevelopmental encephalopathy" (Weinberger, 1995). Some such as Weinberger (1987) consider that all schizophrenia is developmental, while others (e.g. Murray et al., 1985, 1992) suggest that only a proportion of patients have a developmental condition, particularly those with early onset and prominent negative symptoms.

Late developmental theories

A major problem for the early developmental model was to explain why damage presumed to be present since foetal or neonatal life, does not cause psychosis until decades later. The solution proposed was that the crucial lesion(s) could lie silent until the operation of brain maturational processes in adolescence exposed neuronal circuits that are underdeveloped and are not functional in childhood (Benes, 1989; Olney and Farber, 1995; Lipska and Weinberger, 1995). Support for this view came from animal models when Lipska et al. (1993) reported that hippocampal lesions to neonatal rats remain relatively silent until adult life, when the animals develop hyper-response to stress/amphetamines.

Other investigators suggested that if brain maturation in adolescence must be invoked, then perhaps it is abnormal rather than normal, and that the crucial pathological processes might operate during this period. This "late" as opposed to "early" developmental model was initially proposed by Feinberg (1982, 1983) and then later by Keshavan et al. (1994, 1999).

Morphological brain changes identified by brain imaging

Numerous CT studies showed that the brains of patients with schizophrenia are different from those of controls (Johnstone et al., 1976; Weinberger et al., 1983; Lishman, 1983a; Reveley, 1985; Lewis, 1990; Garver, 1997). The lack of evidence of progression led to a consensus that these were static brain changes, reflecting early neurodevelopmental anomalies (Nasrallah, 1990; Jaskiw, 1994; Vita, 1997). Structural MRI confirmed an increase in ventricular size, and subtle but diffuse cortical volume reductions (Johnstone et al., 1976; Lewis, 1990; Harvey et al., 1993; Woodruff and Murray, 1994; Chua and McKenna, 1995; Van Horn et al., 1992). Thus, Zipursky et al. (1992) showed significant reductions in grey matter volumes in most parts of the cerebral cortex, including prefrontal, frontal, temporo-parietal and parieto-occipital regions. Post-mortem studies confirmed the imaging findings of decreased cortical volume (Pakkenberg, 1987; Bogerts, 1999).

Wright et al. (2000) carried out a meta-analysis of 58 MRI studies which compared subjects with schizophrenia with controls, and found the mean cerebral volume was reduced by 2%; the mean total ventricular volume was increased by 26% (greater in lateral ventricles bilaterally); there was a 6% reduction in amygdala (bilaterally); 6% reduction in left and 5% reduction in the right hippocampus; 7% in the left and 5% in the right parahippocampus.

Temporal lobes show the most consistent reductions (Johnstone et al., 1989; DeLisi et al., 1991; Wright et al., 1999, 2000; McCarley et al., 1999; Harrison, 1999) most markedly in the amygdala and hippocampus (Bogerts, 1985, 1990; Suddath et al., 1989; Wright et al., 1999; Sigmundsson et al., 2001). Hirayasu et al. (2001) showed grey matter reductions in the posterior superior temporal gyrus, an area important for language, that were specific to schizophrenia, compared to affective psychosis and normal controls. Studies have less consistently found frontal lobe abnormalities (McCarley et al., 1999). Gur et al. (2000) found reduced prefrontal grey matter particularly in the dorsolateral sector, which related to symptom severity and cognitive function.

The origins of structural brain abnormalities

The associations of ventricular enlargement with obstetric complications (Murray et al., 1985), and with poor premorbid social adjustment (Weinberger et al., 1980), implied that imaging findings pre-dated the illness onset. This view was strengthened by evidence of similar abnormalities in both chronic and first-onset cases (Weinberger et al., 1982; Turner et al., 1986), and in healthy subjects at strong familial risk of the condition (Reveley et al., 1982; Suddath et al., 1990; McDonald et al., 2001). Important support for a neurodevelopmental origin to schizophrenia came from work by Lewis (1990) who reported increased frequency of rare anomalies of brain development such as septal cysts, aqueduct stenosis, agenesis of the corpus callosum and cavum septum pellucidum. Other evidence came from research into cerebral asymmetry. The human brain develops asymmetrically but reduced asymmetry in schizophrenia has been found (Crow et al., 1989; Bruton et al., 1990; Falkai et al., 1993; Bilder et al., 1994, 1999; Bullmore et al., 1994). Given that development of normal brain asymmetry is complete by the middle of the third trimester, these findings support an origin during foetal life.

Minor physical and dermatoglyphic abnormalities are fossilised markers of altered development taking place during foetal life i.e. at the time that the brain (also an ectodermally-derived structure) is undergoing extensive growth. Both have been found in excess in schizophrenia (McGrath et al., 1995; Lane et al., 1997). The relevance of these findings was pointed out by Van Os et al. (2000) who reported an association between dermatoglyphic ridge counts and cerebral structural abnormalities in people with schizophrenia.

Developmental genes

The genetic predisposition to schizophrenia is well established (Cannon et al., 1998; Cardno et al., 1999). The ill members of monozygotic twin pairs discordant for schizophrenia virtually always have larger ventricles than their well cotwins (Reveley et al., 1982; Suddath et al., 1990) but the latter also show more structural brain abnormalities than controls. The Maudsley family study examined families with several affected members and assumed to transmit a high genetic loading (Sharma et al., 1999). Relatives were divided into standard relatives and presumed obligate carriers (relatives who although well themselves, have psychotic offspring as well as psychotic siblings or parents and therefore appear to be transmitting genetic risk). These obligate carriers showed a similar increase in lateral ventricular volume to the patients themselves. Similar findings have been reported by Faraone et al. (2001).

Early environmental hazards

Exposure to pre- and perinatal complications is a risk factor for schizophrenia (Cannon et al., 2000), the association being stronger in those with early onset (Verdoux et al., 1997; Hultman et al., 1999). According to Cannon et al. (2000), the odds of schizophrenia increase linearly with an increasing number of hypoxic-ischaemic complications. Zornberg et al. (2000) also showed an elevated and graded risk of developing schizophrenia associated with hypoxic-ischaemic foetal/neonatal complications. A possible mechanism is that of the excitotoxic effects of hypoxia on the N-methyl-D-aspartate (NMDA) receptor (Olney and Farber, 1995) in the foetal/neonatal brain (Fearon et al., 2000; Cannon et al., 2000). The hippocampus is particularly prone to anoxic damage and Stefanis et al. (1999) showed that hippocampal volume decrement was found in those non-familial patients who had suffered obstetric complications but not in those familial patients without exposure to obstetric complications. Other early risk factors include viral infection, either in utero (Sham et al., 1993; Takei et al., 1996; Verdoux et al., 1997) or postnatally (Rantakillo et al., 1997; Westergaard et al., 1999).

Childhood developmental deviance

Premorbid impairments are found in a proportion of individuals who go on to develop schizophrenia. Around 25–50% of children born to mothers with schizophrenia have poor motor co-ordination in early childhood, or attention and information processing deficits later, suggesting that developmental problems are at least partly inherited (Amminger et al., 1999; Erlenmeyer-Kimling et al., 2000a,b).

Walker et al. (1993) noted more postural and upper limb movement abnormalities in pre-schizophrenic children than in their well siblings; these were most noticeable in the first two years of life (Walker et al., 1996). The 1946 British Birth Cohort Study, which followed up 4746 children for 43 years, demonstrated that the 30 who developed schizophrenia, as a group, had subtly delayed milestones (e.g. walking was delayed by an average of 1.2 months) (Jones et al., 1994). Cannon et al. (2001) have also shown poorer psychomotor and language development in pre-schizophreniform children in a detailed follow-up of a birth cohort from Dunedin, New Zealand.

The study of Jones et al. (1994) just discussed showed more speech problems and lower educational test scores at 8, 11 and 15 in pre-schizophrenic individuals. Indeed, cognitive impairment has been repeatedly reported. Thus, David et al. (1997) examined nearly 50,000 18-year-old males who were conscripted into the Swedish army in 1969–1970, and noted a linear relationship between schizophrenia and IQ with risk gradually increasing as IQ fell at all levels of intellectual ability.

What do histopathological studies suggest?

Loss of Neuropil and Increased Neuronal Density: Post-mortem studies of schizophrenia consistently show reductions in neuronal size, dendritic spine density and length, synaptic proteins and synaptic gene expression (Rajkowska, 1998; Cotter et al., 2001b; Glantz and Lewis, 1997, 2000; Rosoklija et al., 2000; Harrison and Eastwood, 1998; Honer et al., 1999; Perrone-Bizzozero et al., 1996; Akil and Weinberger, 2000; Mirnics et al., 2001).

Smaller neurons with fewer and less elaborate branches would result in a diminution in the amount of neuropil, more compacted cells, and thus increased neuronal density, and this too has been observed in schizophrenia (Selemon et al., 1995). Pathology in subcortical structures is not well established, although evidence for a reduction in the total number of neurons in the dorso-medial thalamus (Pakkenberg et al., 1991; Young et al., 2000; Popken et al., 2000) is convincing. This may reflect reduced numbers of thalamo-cortical projection neurons, and in keeping with this, Lewis and colleagues (2001) recently demonstrated a reduced density of parvalbumin immunoreactive varicosities in the prefrontal cortex. As these varicosities selectively label the axonal terminals of thalamic projection neurons, this could indicate decreased thalamo-cortical connectivity.

Abnormal Pruning of Synapses: The above findings are suggestive of pathology of synapses and their connectivity. The developing brain has a large excess of neurones and axons, which thin out during early development, thus serving to eliminate early errors of connection and to strengthen those that are useful. The relevance of pruning of cortical neurons during adolescence for schizophrenia was introduced by Feinberg (1983), who proposed there may be a fault in progressive synapse elimination. Keshavan and colleagues (1994) used MRS to show that people with schizophrenia show a phosphomonoesterase pattern suggestive of failure of new synapse production and excessive synaptic reduction. This process is postulated to lead to a loss of synaptic connectivity below a critical level (McGlashan and Hoffman, 2000). Murray et al. (1988) and Lewis et al. (1989) postulated immature circuitry laid bare by synaptic pruning, a process which in some brain areas continues until after puberty. Early injury could prevent such processes from occurring, resulting in the perpetuation of anomalous connectivity patterns, which could eventually become operational, resulting in the appearance of the disease.

Early Migration Abnormalities? It is well established that there is a massive neuronal migration, during the second trimester, from the periventricular germinal matrix to the cortex. Three influential papers (Kovelman and Scheibel, 1984; Jakob and Beckmann, 1986; Akbarian et al., 1993, 1996) suggested that this migration might be disturbed in schizophrenia, leading to entorhinal cortex heterotopias and hippocampal neuronal disarray. These findings appeared to provide support for the developmental hypothesis of schizophrenia, but unfortunately replication of the findings has been inconsistent (Harrison et al., 1999; Cotter et al., 1996; Beasley et al., 2001), Indeed, the lack of replication of these findings has been a major factor increasing interest in neurodegeneration.

The case for neurodegeneration

Although neurodevelopmental theory can explain much about liability to schizophrenia, it fails to adequately explain a) the long latent period to onset; b) those cases having their onset in middle or late adult life; or c) the malignantly deteriorating clinical course suffered by some (Murray et al., 1992). The alternative view is that schizophrenia results from an active neurodegenerative process, which is especially prominent during the late teens and early twenties, but continues throughout adult life.

The majority of people with schizophrenia show clinical deterioration but this occurs primarily in the early stages of the illness, is generally confined to the first 5 years, and does not progress in an inexorable manner (Lieberman, 1999; Hafner, 1999). Wyatt (1991) suggested that the likelihood of experiencing deterioration is correlated with the duration and number of periods of active psychosis. Associations between the duration of untreated psychosis and likelihood of developing a more 'malignant' illness seem to support this (Pfohl and Winokur, 1982; Loebel, 1992; Waddington et al., 1995), as do studies of never-medicated patients where the frequency and severity of dyskinetic movement disorders is associated with longer duration of illness (Fenton and McGlashan, 1994; McCreadie et al., 1996). However, Hoff et al. (2000) reported no significant correlations between duration of untreated psychosis and severity of cognitive and structural changes at first episode. Similarly, Verdoux and her colleagues (1997) found that when premorbid characteristics such as childhood function, family history and negative symptoms were taken into account, there was little independent evidence for an adverse effect of duration of untreated psychosis.

There is dispute as to whether there is cognitive decline either in the years immediately before or after the onset of psychosis. Follow-up studies of first onset patients have shown that there is, if anything, a slight improvement, on average, in cognitive function as psychotic symptoms are treated; indeed, improvement in positive symptoms is associated with improvement in cognition abilities (Hoff et al., 1999). IQ doesn't markedly decline in more chronic cases, suggesting that the course of schizophrenia is more consistent with a static encephalopathy than a dementing disorder (Hyde, 1994).

However, there is some evidence that decline in cognitive function in later life tends to be exaggerated in those with schizophrenia (Harvey, 1996; Friedman, 1999). This is not attributable to known dementias (Pantellis, 1992; Harrison, 1995, 1998) or effects of treatment (Baldessarini, 1997). It could be simply that the decline is more noticeable in schizophrenic patients as they have on average less cognitive reserve than the rest of the population.

Late onset schizophrenia (LOS) and very late onset schizophrenia (VLOS) can arise without clinically significant gross structural abnormalities of the brain (Symonds, 1997), but some studies have reported ventricular enlargement, thought to be secondary to white matter change (Howard, 2000). Certainly, it is difficult to attribute such late onset conditions to neurodevelopmental damage (Murray et al., 1992). There is some evidence that these late onset cases have less genetic loading for schizophrenia or exposure to early environmental insult.

Progressive morphometric changes

Structural brain changes occur in late childhood, which reflect processes of late brain maturation thought to play a crucial role in normal cognitive development. These include age-related grey matter volume reductions, greatest in the frontal and parietal convexities (Jernigan et al., 1991). Such changes appear to be particularly prominent in childhood-onset cases of schizophrenia where progressive reduction of temporal lobe structures (Jacobsen et al., 1998) and increasing ventricular enlargement have been reported (Rapoport, 1997).

Several recent follow-up studies of people with schizophrenia have suggested that ventricular enlargement and some changes in the temporal lobes may be progressive (Woods, 1998; DeLisi, 1999; Lieberman, 1999). For example, Pantelis et al. (2001), who looked at a small group of high-risk subjects, claim that those who subsequently developed psychosis showed left-sided reductions in parahippocampal, fusiform and orbitofrontal cortex. They concluded that this change may start in the prodrome before frank symptoms are expressed. In a study of first onset cases, Cahn et al. (2001) found 1.2% decrease in grey and 7.5% increase in lateral ventricular volume one year after onset.

Perhaps the most convincing evidence comes from DeLisi et al. (1995) who carried out within-subject serial volumetric MR1 examinations in first onset schizophrenic patients and age-matched controls. They found an increased rate of atrophy in the left temporal lobe; their 4 year findings showed a significantly greater rate of change in both cerebral hemispheres and left ventricular enlargement (DeLisi, 1997b). They concluded that "this reflects an ongoing degenerative process" (DeLisi, 1999). Progressive regional changes reported have included significant volume reductions in the frontal lobes at 3 year (Gur et al., 1998) and 5 year follow up (Madsen, 1999). Mathalon et al. (2001) claimed that patients with chronic schizophrenia exhibited accelerated fronto-temporal cortical grey matter reductions and sulcal and lateral ventricle enlargement in a 4 year controlled follow-up; greater clinical severity was associated with faster rates of change. Gharaibeh et al. (2000), in a 3–5 year follow-up, also claimed to find significant change though this could have been a treatment effect. However, Lieberman et al. (2001), in a 6 year follow-up, observed no significant reduction in cortical and hippocampal volumes, and no overall change in ventricular size.

Several authors have suggested that there may be differences between good and poor outcome patients. Nair et al. (1997) identified two subgroups in a 2–3 year follow-up; those with static and those with progressive ventricular enlargement; neither was accounted for by co-morbid drug/alcohol misuse, compliance or clinical correlates. Davis et al. (1998) found that a so-called "Kraepelinian" subgroup of severe patients showed ventricular enlargement over 4 year period compared with non-Kraepelinian people with schizophrenia and controls. However, Falke et al. (2000) who looked for subcortical degeneration of poor outcome patients found no progressive changes in the thalamus or caudate nuclei.

Is there neuropathological evidence of degeneration?

The reductions in neuronal size and in the synaptic and dendritic components of the cortex, which we discussed earlier (Harrison, 1999; Mirnicks et al., 2001; Cotter et al., 2001), are compatible with a neurodegenerative process. However, there is no direct evidence that these or the findings of volume decrements on follow-up MRI studies, reflect neurodegeneration (see reviews by Bogerts, 1993; Harrison, 1999). There remains little neuropathological evidence of postmaturational neural injury (Arnold, 1998, 1999; Arnold et al., 1998). Indeed, even among a cohort of elderly schizophrenic subjects showing cognitive decline there was no evidence for excess Alzheimers disease pathology or degenerative disorders generally (Purohit et al., 1998).

The critical abnormalities of neuronal loss, senile plaques, neurofibrillary tangles and gliosis are generally thought to be absent in schizophrenia. Gliosis, a sign of past inflammation (Kreutzberg et al., 1997) was reported by Stevens (1982) in around 70% of cases studied, mainly in the periventricular, diencephalic and basal forebrain structures. Similar observations were made by Nieto and Escobar (1972), and raised the possibility of an inflammatory process. However, subsequent studies failed to replicate these findings (Roberts et al., 1986, 1987; Stevens et al., 1988; Arnold et al., 1996). In Bruton et al's (1990) carefully controlled investigation, the excess gliosis disappeared after excluding patients with Alzheimer changes, cerebrovascular disease and focal pathologies. Thus, gliosis is not an intrinsic feature of schizophrenia.

However, since progression might not reflect degeneration, the absence of gliosis doesn't exclude all forms of neuropathological progression. Indeed, gliosis is not always demonstrable after post-natal injury, and it does not accompany apoptosis (Harrison, 1999). Apoptosis is programmed cell death; the processes of neuropil turnover, maintenance and elimination (Kerr, 1972). The apoptotic cascade is an intracellular death program released from inhibition by genetically encoded protease activation of caspases. The process occurs normally, without associated inflammation, in early development and with ageing (Woods, 1998). Its inappropriate activation leads to pathological loss of cells, and is thought to play a part in chronic degenerative disorders (Gibson, 2001), without structural changes being observable neuropathologically. To date, a single study has demonstrated reduced levels of Bcl-2, a component of the antiapoptotic pathway, in the cortex in schizophrenia (Jarskog et al., 2000). This is in keeping with the observed reductions in neuronal and synapto-dendritic components in the disorder, but the problem with implicating the pro-apoptotic pathway in schizophrenia is that apoptosis occurs over a rapid timescale. If this pathway were involved in schizophrenia, one would expect evidence of cortical neuronal loss, and this has not been described (Harrison, 1999).

Is there a role for glucocorticoids?

Could glucocorticoid-related neurotoxicity explain the histopathological changes found in schizophrenia? Hyperactivity of the hypothalamic pituitary adrenal (HPA) axis is typically involved in the pathogenesis of mood disorder (Pariante and Miller, 2001). Furthermore, reduced glucocorticoid related gene expression has been recently described in the frontal cortex in both schizophrenia and major depression (Webster et al., 2000) providing the first firm evidence that HPA axis abnormalities are a feature of schizophrenia.

Several lines of investigation raise the possibility that glucocorticoid-related neurotoxicity may be implicated in both depression and schizophrenia. Firstly, in vitro investigations have shown that high levels of glucocorticoid hormones result in reduced neuronal volume and dendritic arborisation (Sapolsky, 2000a,b), and these changes have been observed in both disorders. Secondly, elevated plasma glucocorticoid levels are associated with hippocampal volume reductions such as those claimed to occur during the first psychotic episode (Pantellis et al., 2000; Lawrie et al., 2000). Finally, the functional effect of glucocorticoids on reducing hippocampal glial cell activation and proliferation (Crossin et al., 1997) mirrors the glial deficit observed in major depression, bipolar disorder and possibly schizophrenia. These data raise the possibility that some of the brain changes seen in schizophrenia may be secondary to the depressive symptoms and the associated elevation in glucocorticoid levels that accompany the illnesses.

Conclusion

It is indisputable that there is a developmental component to schizophrenia. Dysplastic neural development could account not only for many of the clinical characteristics of the illness but also for the loss of neurophil seen in postmortem studies and the dysfunctional circuitry seen in functional imaging studies (Bullmore et al., 1997). However, we cannot yet say whether schizophrenia results simply from aberrant development or whether additional neurodegenerative processes are initiated at, or shortly before, the onset of psychosis. In recent years, several hypotheses have been put forward to link both developmental and degenerative theories. McCarley (1999) suggests a two "hit" hypothesis while Keshavan (1999) and Velakoulis et al. (2000) both suggest three "hits" are necessary. The latter, for example, hypothesise that an early developmental lesion leads to vulnerability, with further insults at transition to illness and progression to chronic, persistent illness.

Although schizophrenia is not "neurodegenerative" in the traditional sense, some MRI studies suggest that there may be reductions in the volume of certain brain structures at, or just before, the onset of psychosis and continuing for several years thereafter. These changes are compatible with either late maturational or degenerative processes and, although there is relatively little direct evidence of the latter from neuropathology, glucocorticoid neurotoxicity is being investigated as a possible explanatory process. Nevertheless, if there are such changes in the first five years following onset of psychosis, how is it that at the same time neuropsychological studies show that cognitive function is either static or improving? Any plausible degenerative theory requires to explain this curious paradox.

References

Akbarian S, Jones EG (1996) Developmental abnormalities of the prefrontal cortex in schizophrenia. Biol Psychiatry 39: 200

Akbarian S, Bunney WE Jr, Potkin SG, Wigal S, Hagman JO, Sandman CA, Jones EG (1993) Altered distribution of nicotinamideadenine dinucleotide phosphate-diaphorase cells in frontal lobe of schizophrenics implies disturbances of cortical development. Arch Gen Psychiatry 50: 169–177

Akil M, Weinberger DR (2000) Gliosis and its implications for the disease process. In: Harrison P, Roberts G (eds) The neuropathology of schizophrenia, 1st edn. Oxford University Press, New York, pp 137–145

Amminger GP, Pape S, Rock D, Roberts SA, Ott SL, Squires-Wheeler E, Kestenbaum C, Erlenmeyer-Kimling L (1999) Relationship between childhood behavioral disturbance and later schizophrenia in the New York High-Risk Project. Am J Psychiatry 156: 525–530

Arnold SE (1999) Cognition and neuropathology in schizophrenia. Acta Psychiatr Scand [Suppl] 99(395): 41–50

Arnold SE (2001) Contributions of neuropathology to understanding schizophrenia in late life. Harvard Rev Psychiatry 9(2): 69–76

Arnold SE, Trojanowski JO (1996) Recent advances in defining the neuropathology of schizophrenia. Acta Neuropathol 92: 217–231

Arnold SE, Trojanowski JQ, Gur RE, Blackwell P, Han L-Y, Choi C (1998) Absence of neurodegeneration and neural injury in the cerebral cortex in a sample of elderly patients with schizophrenia. Arch Gen Psychiatry 55(3): 225–232

Baldessarini RJ, Hegarty JD, Bird ED, Benes FM (1997) Meta-analysis of postmortem studies of Alzeimer's disease-like neuropathology in schizophrenia. Am J Psychiatry 154(6): 861–863

Beasley C, Cotter D, Khan N, Pollard C, Sheppard P, Varndell I, Lovestone S, Anderton B, Everall I (2001) Glycogen synthase kinase-3(beta) immunoreactivity is reduced in the prefrontal cortex in schizophrenia. Neurosci Lett 302(2–3): 117–120

Benes FM (1989) Myelination of cortical-hippocampal relays during late adolescence. Schizophr Bull 15: 585–593

Bilder RM, Wu H, Bogerts B, Degreef G, Ashtari M, Alvir JMJ, Snyder P, Lieberman JA (1994) Absence of regional hemispheric volume asymmetries in first-episode schizophrenia. Am J Psychiatry 151: 1437–1447

Bilder RM, Wu H, Bogerts B, Ashtari M, Robinson D, Woerner M, Lieberman JA, Degreef G (1999) Cerebral volume asymmetries in schizophrenia and mood disorders: a quantitative magnetic resonance imaging study. Int J Psychophysiol 34(3): 197–205

Bogerts B (1993) Recent advances in the neuropathology of schizophrenia. Schizophr Bull 19(2): 431–445

Bogerts B (1999) The neuropathology of schizophrenic diseases: historical aspects and present knowledge. Eur Arch Psychiatry Clin N 249: 2–13

Bogerts B, Meertz E, Bausch-Schofeldt R (1985) Basal ganglia and limbic system pathology in schizophrenia: a morphometric study of brain volume and shrinkage. Arch Gen Psychiatry 42: 784–791

Bogerts B, Ashtari M, Degreef G, Alvir JM, Bilder RM, Lieberman JA (1990) Reduced temporal limbic structure volumes on magnetic resonance images in first episode schizophrenia. Psychiat Res: Neuroimaging Sect 35: 1–13

Bramon E, Kelly J, Van Os J, Murray RM (2001) The cascade of increasingly deviant development that culminates in the onset of schizophrenia. Neurosci News 4(1): 5–19

Bruton CJ, Crow TJ, Frith CD, Johnstone EC, Owens DG, Roberts GW (1990) Schizophrenia and the brain: a prospective clinico-neuropathological study. Psychol Med 20: 285–304

Bullmore E, Brammer M, Harvey I, Murray R, Ron M (1995) Cerebral hemispheric-asymmetry revisited — effects of handedness, gender and schizophrenia measured by radius of gyration in magnetic-resonance images. Psychol Med 25(2): 349–363

Bullmore ET, Frangou S, Murray RM (1997) The dysplastic net hypothesis: an integration of developmental and dysconnectivity theories of schizophrenia. Schizophr Res 28: 143–156

Cahn W, Hulshoff Pol HE, Lems EB, van Haren NE, Schnack HG, van der Linden JA, Schothorst PF, van Engeland H, Kahn RS (2002) Brain volume changes in first-episode schizophrenia: a one-year follow-up study (submitted)

Cannon TD, Kaprio J, Lonnqvist J, Huttunen M, Koskenvuo M (1998) The genetic epidemiology of schizophrenia in a Finnish twin cohort — a population-based modeling study. Arch Gen Psychiatry 55: 67–74

Cannon TD, Rosso IM, Hollister JM, Bearden CE, Sanchez LE, Hadley T (2000) A prospective cohort study of genetic and perinatal influences in the etiology of schizophrenia. Schizophr Bull 26(2): 351–366

Cardno AG, Marshall EJ, Cold B, Macdonald AM, Ribchester TR, Davies NJ, Venturi P, Jones LA, Lewis SW, Sham PC, Gottesman II, Farmer AE, McGuffin P, Reveley AM, Murray RM (1999) Heritability estimates for psychotic disorders — The Maudsley Twin psychosis series. Arch Gen Psychiatry 56: 162–168

Chua SE, McKenna PJ (1995) Schizophrenia — a brain disease — a critical-review of structural and functional cerebral abnormality in the disorder. Br J Psychiatry 166: 563–582

Clouston T (1891) The neuroses of development. Oliver & Boyd, Edinburgh

Cotter D, Kerwin R, Doshi R, Everall I (1997) Alterations in hippocampal non-phosphorylated MAP2 expression in schizophrenia. Brain Res 765(2): 238–246

Cotter D, Mackay D, Landau S, Kerwin D, Everall I (2001) Glial cell loss and reduced neuronal size in the anterior cingulate cortex in major depressive disorder. Arch Gen Psychiatry 58: 545–553

Cotter D, Pariante CM, Rajkowska G (2001) Glial pathology in major psychiatric disorders. In: Belmaker RH, Agam G (eds) The postmortem brain in psychiatric research. Kluwer Academic Publishers (in press)

Crossin KL, Tai M-H, Krushel LA, Mauro VP, Edelman GM (1997) Glucocorticoid receptor pathways are involved in the inhibition of astrocyte proliferation. Proc Natl Acad Sci USA 94(6): 2687–2692

Crow TJ, Ball J, Bloom SR, Brown R, Bruton CJ, Colter N, Frith CD, Johnstone EC, Owens DG, Roberts GW (1989) Schizophrenia as an anomaly of development of cerebral asymmetry. A postmortem study and a proposal concerning the genetic-basis of the disease. Arch Gen Psychiatry 46(12): 1145–1150

David AS, Malmberg A, Brandt L, Allebeck P, Lewis G (1997) IQ and risk for schizophrenia: a population-based cohort study. Psych Med 27: 1311–1323

Davis K-L, Buchsbaum MS, Shihabuddin L, Spiegel-Cohen J, Metzger M, Frecska E, Keefe RS, Powchik P (1998) Ventricular enlargement in poor-outcome schizophrenia. Biol Psychiatry 43: 783–793

DeLisi L (1999) Defining the course of brain structural change and plasticity in schizophrenia. Psychiat Res: Neuroimaging Sect 92: 1–9

DeLisi LE, Hoff AL, Schwartz JE, Shields GW, Halthore SN, Gupta SM, Henn FA, Anand AK (1991) Brain morphology in first-episode schizophrenic-like psychotic patients: a quantitative magnetic resonance imaging study. Biol Psychiatry 29: 159–175

DeLisi LE, Tew W, Xie S-K, Hoff AL, Sakuma M, Kushner M, Lee G, Shedlack K, Smith AM, Grimson R (1995) A prospective follow-up study of brain morphology and cognition in lst episode schizophrenic patients. Biol Psychiatry 38: 349–360

DeLisi LE, Sakurna M, Tew W, Kushner M, Hoff AL, Grimson R (1997) Schizophrenia as a chronic active brain process: a study of progressive brain structural change subsequent to the onset of schizophrenia. Psychiat Res: Neuroimaging 74: 129–140

Duman RS, Heninger GR, Nestler EJ (1997) A molecular and cellular theory of depression. Arch Gen Psychiatry 54(7): 597–606

Erlenmeyer-Kimling L (2000a) Neurobehavioral deficits in offspring of schizophrenic parents: liability indicators and predictors of illness. Am J Med Genet 97(1): 65–71

Erlenmeyer-Kimling L, Rock D, Roberts SA, Janal M, Kestenbaum C, Cornblatt B, Adamo UH, Gottesman II (2000b) Attention, memory, and motor skills as childhood predictors of schizophrenia-related psychoses: the New York high-risk project. Am J Psychiatry 157(9): 1416–1422

Falkai P, Bogerts B, Greve B, Pfeiffer U, Machus B, Folsch-Reetz B, Majtenyi C, Ovary I (1992) Loss of sylvian fissure asymmetry in schizophrenia. A quantitative post mortem study. Schizophr Res 7(1): 23–32

Falke E, Han L-Y, Arnold SE (2000) Absence of neurodegeneration in the thalamus and caudate of elderly patients with schizophrenia. Psychiatry Res 93(2): 103–110

Faraone SV, Green AI, Seidman LJ, Tsuang MT (2001) "Schizotaxia": clinical implications and new directions for research. Schizophr Bull 27: 1–18

Fearon P, Cotter D, Murray R (2000) Is the association between obstetric complications and schizophrenia mediated by glutamatergic excitotoxic damage in the fetal/neonatal brain? In: Reveley AM, Deakin J (eds) The psychopharmacology of schizophrenia, 1 ed. Arnold, London, pp 21–40

Feinberg I (1982–1983) Schizophrenia: caused by a fault in programmed synaptic elimination during adolescence. J Psychiat Res 17: 319–334

Fenton WS, McGlashan TH (1994) Antecedents, symptom progression, and long-term outcome of the deficit syndrome in schizophrenia. Am J Psychiatry 151: 351–356

Foong J, Symms MR, Barker GJ, Maier M, Woermann FG, Miller DH, Ron MA (2001) Neuropathological abnormalities in schizophrenia: evidence from magnetization transfer imaging. Brain 124: 882–892

Friedman JI, Harvey PD, Kemether E, Byne W, Davis KL (1999) Cognitive and functional changes with aging in schizophrenia. Biol Psychiatry 46(7): 921–928

Garver DL (1997) The aetiologic heterogeneity of schizophrenia: review and perspective. Harvard Rev Psychiatry 4: 317–327

Gharaibeh WS, Rohlf FJ, Slice DE, DeLisi LE (2000) A geometric morphometric assessment of change in midline brain structural shape following a first episode of schizophrenia. Biol Psychiatry 48(5): 398–405

Gibson R (2001) Does apotosis have a role in neurodegeneration? BMJ 322: 1539–1540

Glantz LA, Lewis DA (1997) Reduction of synaptophysin immunoreactivity in the prefrontal cortex of subjects with schizophrenia: regional and diagnostic specificity. Arch Gen Psychiatry 54(7): 660–669

Glantz LA, Lewis DA (2000) Decreased dendritic spine density on prefrontal cortical pyramidal neurons in schizophrenia. Arch Gen Psychiatry 57: 65–73

Gur RE, Cowell P, Turetsky BI, Gallacher N, Cannon T, Bilker W, et al (1998) A follow-up magnetic resonance imaging study of schizophrenia: relationship of neuroanatomical changes to clinical and neurobehavioral measures. Arch Gen Psychiatry 55: 145–152

Gur RE, Cowell PE, Latshaw A, Turetsky BI, Grossman RI, Arnold SE, Bilker WB, Gur RC (2000) Reduced dorsal and orbital prefrontal gray matter volumes in schizophrenia. Arch Gen Psychiatry 57(8): 761–768

Hafner H, Ander Heiden W (1999) The course of schizophrenia in the light of modern follow-up studies: the ABC and WHO studies. Eur Arch Psychiatry Clin N 249 [Suppl 4]: IV14–IV26

Harrison PJ (1995) On the neuropathology of schizophrenia and its dementia: neurodevelopmental, neurodegenerative or both? Neurodegeneration 4(1): 1–12

Harrison PJ (1999) The neuropathology of schizophrenia — a critical review of the data and their interpretation. Brain 122: 593–624

Harrison PJ, Eastwood SL (1998) Preferential involvement of excitatory neurons in medial temporal lobe in schizophrenia. Lancet 352(9141): 1669–1673

Harvey L, Ron MA, Du Boulay G, Wicks D, Lewis SW, Murray RM (1993) Reduction of cortical volume in schizophrenia on magnetic resonance imaging. Psychol Med 23: 591–604

Harvey PD, Lombardi J, Leibman M, White L, Parrella M, Powchik P, Mohs RC, Davidson M (1996) Performance of chronic schizophrenic patients on cognitive neuropsychological measures sensitive to dementia. Int J Geriatr Psych 11(7): 621–627

Hirayasu Y, McCarley RW, Salisbury DF, Tanaka S, Jun Soo Kwon, Frumin M, Snyderman D, Yurgelun-Todd D, Kikinis R, Jolesz FA, Shenton ME (2000) Planum Temporale and Heschl gyrus volume reduction in schizophrenia: a magnetic resonance imaging study of first-episode patients. Arch Gen Psychiatry 57(7): 692–699

Hirayasu Y, Tanaka S, Shenton ME, Salisbury DF, DeSantis MA, Levitt JJ, Wible C, Yurgelun-Todd D, Kikinis R, Jolesz FA, McCarley RW (2001) Prefrontal gray matter volume reduction in first episode schizophrenia. Cereb Cortex 11(4): 374–381

Hoff Al, Sakuma M, Wieneke M, Horon R, Kushner M, DeLisi L (1999) Longitudinal neuropsychological follow-up study of patients with first-episode schizophrenia. Am J Psychiatry 156(9): 1336–1341

Hoff AL, Sakuma M, Razi K, Heydebrand G, Csernansky JG, DeLisi LE (2000) Lack of association between duration of untreated illness and severity of cognitive and structural brain deficits at the first episode of schizophrenia. Am J Psychiatry 157(11): 1824–1828

Honer WG, Falkai P, Chen C, Arango V, Mann JJ, Dwork AJ (1999) Synaptic and plasticity-associated proteins in anterior frontal cortex in severe mental illness. Neuroscience 91(4): 1247–1255

Howard R, Rabins P, Seeman M, Jeste DV (2000) Late-onset schizophrenia and very-late-onset schizophrenia-like psychosis: an international consensus. Am J Psychiatry 157(2): 172–178

Hultman CM, Sparen P, Takei N, Murray RM, Cnattingius S (1999) Prenatal and perinatal risk factors for schizophrenia, affective psychosis, and reactive psychosis of early onset: case-control study. Br Med J 318: 421–426

Hyde TM, Nawroz S, Goldberg TE, Bigelow LB, Strong D, Ostrem JL, Weinberger DR, Kleinman JE (1994) Is there cognitive decline in schizophrenia? A cross-sectional study. Br J Psychiatry 164: 494–500

Jacobsen LK, Giedd JX, Castellanos X, Vaituzis AC, Hamburger SD, Kurnra S, Lenane MC, Rapoport J (1998) Progressive reduction of temporal lobe structures in childhood-onset schizophrenia. Am J Psychiatry 155: 678–685

Jakob H, Beckmann H (1986) Prenatal developmental disturbances in the limbic allocortex in schizophrenia. J Neural Transm 65: 303–326

Jarskog LF, Gilmore JH, Selinger ES, Lieberman JA (2000) Cortical Bcl-2 protein expression and apoptotic regulation in schizophrenia. Biol Psychiatry 48(7): 641–650

Jaskiw GE, Juliano DM, Goldberg TE, Hertzman M, Urow-Hamell E, Weinberger DR (1994) Cerebral ventricular enlargement in schizophreniform disorder does not progress: a seven year follow-up study. Schizophr Res 14: 23–28

Jernigan TIL, Trauner DA, Hesselink JR, Talial PA (1991) Maturation of human cerebrum observed in vivo during adolescence. Brain 114: 2037–2049

Johnstone EC, Crow TJ, Frith CD, Husband J, Kreel L (1976) Cerebral ventricular size and cognitive impairment in chronic schizophrenia. Lancet ii: 924–926

Johnstone EC, Owens DGC, Bydder GM, Colter N, Crow TJ, Frith CD (1989) The spectrum of structural brain changes in schizophrenia — age of onset as a predictor of cognitive and clinical impairments and their cerebral correlates. Psychol Med 19: 91–103

Jones P, Rodgers B, Murray R, Marmot M (1994) Child developmental risk-factors for adult schizophrenia in the British 1946 Birth Cohort. Lancet 344: 1398–1402

Kerr JF, Wyllie AH, Currie AR (1972) Apoptosis: a basic biological phenomenon with wide ranging implications in tissue kinetics. Br J Cancer 26: 239–257

Keshavan MS (1999) Development, disease and degeneration in schizophrenia: a unitary pathophysiological model. J Psychiat Res 33(6): 513–521

Keshavan MS, Anderson S, Pettegrew JW (1994) Is schizophrenia due to excessive synaptic pruning in the prefrontal cortex? The Feinberg hypothesis revisited. J Psychiatr Res 28: 239–265

Kovelman J, Scheibel A (1984) A neurobiological correlate of schizophrenia. Biol Psychiatry 19: 1601–1621

Kraepelin E (1896) Dementia praecox. The clinical roots of the schizophrenia concept, 5th ed. Cambridge University Press, Leipzig, pp 426–441

Kreutzberg GW (1996) Microglia: a sensor for pathological events in the CNS. TINS 19: 312–318

Lane A, Kinsella A, Murphy P, Byrne M, Keenan J, Colgan K, Cassidy B, Sheppard N, Horgan R, Waddington JL, Larkin C, O'Callaghan E (1997) The anthropometric assessment of dysmorphic features in schizophrenia as an index of its developmental origins. Psychol Med 27(5): 1155–1164

Lawrie SM, Whalley H, Byrne M, Miller P, Best JJK, Johnstone E (2000) Brain structure change and psychopathology in subjects at high risk of schizophrenia. Schizophr Res 41(1): 11

Lewis DA, Cruz DA, Melchitzky DS, Pierri JN (2001) Lamina-specific deficits in parvalbumin-immunoreactive varicosities in the prefrontal cortex of subjects with schizophrenia: evidence for fewer projections from the thalamus. Am J Psychiatry 158(9): 1411–1422

Lewis S (1990) Computerised topography in schizophrenia 15 years on. Br J Psychiatry 157: 16–24

Lewis SW, Owen MJ, Murray RM (1989) Obstetric complications and schizophrenia: methodology and mechanisms. Oxford University Press, New York

Lieberman J, Chakos M, Wu H, Alvir J, Hoffman E, Robinson D, Bilder R (2001) Longitudinal study of brain morphology in first-episode schizophrenia. Biol Psychiatry 49(6): 487–499

Lieberman JA (1999) Is schizophrenia a neurodegenerative disorder? A clinical and neurobiological perspective. Biol Psychiatry 46: 729–739

Lipska BK, Weinberger DR (1995) Genetic-variation in vulnerability to the behavioral-effects of neonatal hippocampal damage in rats. Proc Natl Acad Sci USA 92: 8906–8910

Lipska BK, Jaskiw GE, Weinberger DR (1993) Postpubertal emergence of hyper-responsiveness to stress and to amphetamine after neonatal excitotoxic hippocampal damage — a potential animal-model of schizophrenia. Neuropsychopharmacol 9: 67–75

Lishman WA (1983) The apparatus of mind: brain structure and function in mental disorder. Psychosomatics 24: 699–720

Loebel AD, Lieberman JA, Alvir JMJ, Mayerhoff DI, Geisler SH, Szymanski SR (1992) Duration of psychosis and outcome in first-episode schizophrenia. Am J Psychiatry 149: 1183–1188

Madsen A, Karle A, Rubin P, Cortsen M, Andersen H, Hemmingsen R (1999) Progressive atrophy of the frontal lobes in first-episode schizophrenia: interaction with clinical course and neuroleptic treatment. Acta Psychiatr Scand 100: 367–374

Mathalon DH, Sullivan EV, Lim KO, Pfefferbaum A (2001) Progressive brain volume changes and the clinical course of schizophrenia in men: a longitudinal magnetic resonance imaging study. Arch Gen Psychiatry 58(2): 148–157

McCarley RW, Wible CG, Frumin M, Hirayasu Y, Fischer IA, Shenton ME (1999) MRI anatomy of schizophrenia. Biol Psychiatry 45: 1085–1098

McCreadie RG, Thara R, Kamath S, Padmavathy R, Latha S, Mathrubootham N, et al (1996) Abnormal movements in never-medicated Indian patients with schizophrenia. Br J Psychiatry 168: 221–226

McDonald C, Chitnis X, Wright IC, Bullmore ET, Suckling J, Sharma T, Murray RM (2001) Grey matter volume deficits of temporal and frontal regions in schizophrenia. Schizophr Res 49(1–2): 161–161

McGlashan TH, Hoffman RE (2000) Schizophrenia as a disorder of developmentally reduced synaptic connectivity. Arch Gen Psychiatry 57: 637–648

McGrath JJ, van Os J, Hoyos C, Jones PB, Harvey I, Murray RM (1995) Minor physical anomalies in psychoses: associations with clinical and putative aetiological variables. Schizophr Res 18: 9–20

Mirnics K, Middleton FA, Marquez A, Lewis DA, Levitt P (2000) Molecular characterization of schizophrenia viewed by microarray analysis of gene expression in prefrontal cortex. Neuron 28(1): 53–67
Murray RM, Lewis SW (1987) Is schizophrenia a neurodevelopmental disorder? Br Med J (Clin Res Ed) 295: 681–682
Murray RM, Lewis SW, Reveley AM (1985) Towards an aetiological classification of schizophrenia. Lancet i: 1023–1026
Murray RM, Lewis SW, Owen MJ (1988) The neurodevelopmental origins of dementia praecox. In: McGuffin P, Bebbington P (eds) Schizophrenia — the major issues. Heinemann, London, pp 90–107
Murray RM, Ocallaghan E, Castle DJ, Lewis SW (1992) A neurodevelopmental approach to the classification of schizophrenia. Schizophr Bull 18: 319–332
Nair TR, Christensen JD, Kingsbury S1, Kumar NG, Terry WM, Garver DL (1997) Progression of cerebroventricular enlargement and the subtyping of schizophrenia. Psychiat Res (Neuroimaging) 74: 141–150
Nasrallah HA (1990) Brain structure and function in schizophrenia: evidence for fetal neurodevelopmental impairment. Curr Opin Psychiatry 3(1): 75–78
Nieto D, Escobar A (1972) Major psychoses. In: Minkler J (ed) Pathology of the nervous system, vol. 3. McGraw Hill, New York, pp 2654–2665
Pakkenberg B (1987) Post-mortem study of chronic schizophrenic brains. Br J Psychiatry 151: 744–752
Pakkenberg B, Moller A, Gunclersen HJG, Mouritzen Dam A (1991) The absolute number of nerve cells in substantia nigra in normal subjects and in patients with Parkinson's disease estimated with an unbiased stereoiogical method. J Neurol Neurosurg Psychiatry 54: 30–33
Pantelis C, Barnes TR, Nelson HE (1992) Is the concept of frontal-subcortical dementia relevant to schizophrenia? Br J Psychiatry 160: 442–460
Pantelis C, Velakoulis D, McCorry P, Suckling J, Wood SJ, Phillips L, Yung A, Bullmore ET, Brewer W, Soulsby B, Desmond P, McGuire P (2001) Left medial temporal volume reduction occurs during the transition from high-risk to first episode psychosis. Schizophr Res 41(1): 35
Pariante CM, Miller AH (2001) Glucocorticoid receptors in major depression: relevance to pathophysiology and treatment. Biol Psychiatry 49(5): 391–404
Perrone-Bizzozero NI, Sowers AC, Bird ED, Benowitz LI, Ivins KJ, Neve RL (1996) Levels of the growth-associated protein GAP-43 are selectively increased in association cortices in schizophrenia. Proc Natl Acad Sci USA 93(24): 14182–14187
Pfohl B, Winokur G (1982) The evolution of symptoms in institutionialized hebephrenic/catatonic schizophrenics. Br J Psychiatry 141: 567–572
Popken GJ, Bunney WE Jr, Potkin SG, Jones EG (2000) Subnucleus-specific loss of neurons in medial thalamus of schizophrenics. Proc Natl Acad Sci USA 97(16): 9276–9280
Purohit DP, Perl DP, Haroutunian V, Powchik P, Davidson M, Davis KL (1998) Alzheimer disease and related neurodegenerative diseases in elderly patients with schizophrenia: a postmortem neuropathologic study of 100 cases. Arch Gen Psychiatry 55(3): 205–211
Rajkowska G, Selemon LD, Goldman-Rakic PS (1998) Neuronal and glial somal size in the prefrontal cortex: a post-mortem morphometric study of schizophrenia and Huntington disease. Arch Gen Psychiatry 55: 215–224
Rantakallio P, Jones P, Moring J, VonWendt L (1997) Association between central nervous system infections during childhood and adult onset schizophrenia and other psychoses: a 28-year follow-up. Int J Epidemiol 26: 837–843
Rapoport JL, Giedd L, Kurnra S, Jacobsen L, Smith A, Lee P, Nelson L, Hamburger S (1997) Childhood-onset schizophrenia: progressive ventricular change during adolescence. Arch Gen Psychiatry 54: 897–903
Reveley AM, Reveley MA, Clifford CA, Murray RM (1982) Cerebral ventricular size in twins discordant for schizophrenia. Lancet i(8271): 540–541

Reveley MA (1985) CT scans in schizophrenia. Br J Psychiatry 146: 367–371

Roberts GW, Cotter N, Lofthouse R, Bogerts B, Zech M, Crow TJ (1986) Gliosis in schizophrenia: a survey. Biol Psychiatry 21: 1043–1050

Roberts GW, Cotter N, Lofthouse R, Johnstone EC, Crow TJ (1987) Is there gliosis in schizophrenia? Investigation of the temporal lobe. Biol Psychiatry 22: 1459–1468

Rosoklija G, Toomayan G, Ellis SP, Keilp J, Mann JJ, Latov N, Hays AP, Dwork AJ (2000) Structural abnormalities of subicular dendrites in subjects with schizophrenia and mood disorders: preliminary findings. Arch Gen Psychiatry 57(4): 349–356

Saijo T, Abe T, Someya Y, Sassa T, Sudo Y, Suhara T, Shuno T, Asai K, Okubo Y (2001) Ten year progressive ventricular enlargement in schizophrenia: an MRI morphometrical study. Psychiatry Clin Neurosci 55(1): 41–47

Sapolsky RM (2000a) Glucocorticoids and hippocampal atrophy in neuropsychiatric disorders. Arch Gen Psychiatry 57(10): 925–935

Sapolsky RM (2000b) The possibility of neurotoxicity in the hippocampus in major depression: a primer on neuron death. Biol Psychiatry 48(8): 755–765

Schulsinger F, Parnas J, Petersen ET (1984) Cerebral ventricular size in the offspring of schizophrenic mothers — a preliminary-study. Arch Gen Psychiatry 41: 602–606

Selemon LD, Rajkowska G, Goldman-Rakic PS (1995) Abnormally high neuronal density in the schizophrenic cortex: a morphometric analysis of prefrontal area 9 and occipital area 17. Arch Gen Psychiatry 52: 805–818

Sham PC, Maclean CJ, Kendler KS (1993) Risk of schizophrenia and age difference with older siblings — evidence for a maternal viral-infection hypothesis. Br J Psychiatry 163: 627–633

Sharma T, Lancaster E, Sigmundsson T, Lewis S, Takei N, Gurling H, Barta P, Pearlson G, Murray R (1999) Lack of normal pattern of cerebral asymmetry in familial schizophrenic patients and their relatives — The Maudsley Family Study. Schizophr Res 40: 111–120

Sigmundsson T, Suckling J, Maier M, Williams SCR, Bullmore ET, Greenwood KE, Fukuda R, Ron MA, Toone BK (2001) Structural abnormalities in frontal, temporal, and limbic regions and interconnecting white matter tracts in schizophrenic patients with prominent negative symptoms. Am J Psychiatry 158: 234–243

Stefanis N, Frangou S, Yakeley J, Sharma T, O'Connell P, Morgan K, Sigmudsson T, Taylor M, Murray RM (1999) Hippocampal volume reduction in schizophrenia: effects of genetic risk and pregnancy and birth complications. Biol Psychiatry 46: 697–702

Stevens CD, Altshuler LL, Bogerts B, Falkai P (1988) Quantitative study of gliosis in schizophrenia and Huntington's chorea. Biol Psychiatry 24(6): 697–700

Stevens JR (1982) Neuropathology of schizophrenia. Arch Gen Psychiatry 39: 1131–1139

Suddath RL, Casanova MF, Goldberg TE, Daniel DG, Kelsoe Jr JR, Weinberger DR (1989) Temporal lobe pathology in schizophrenia: a quantitative magnetic resonance imaging study. Am J Psychiatry 146(4): 464–472

Suddath RL, Christison GW, Torrey EF, Casanova MF, Weinberger DR (1990) Anatomical abnormalities in the brain of monozygotic twins discordant for schizophrenia. N Engl J Med 322: 789–794

Symonds LL, Olichney JM, Jernigan TL, Corey-Bloom J, Healy JF, Jeste DV (1997) Lack of clinically significant gross structural abnormalities in MRIs of older patients with schizophrenia and related psychoses. J Neuropsych Clin N 9(2): 251–258

Takei N, Mortensen PB, Klaening U, Murray RM, Sham PC, O'Callaghan E, Munk-Jorgensen P (1996) Relationship between in utero exposure to influenza epidemics and risk of schizophrenia in Denmark. Biol Psychiatry 40: 817–824

Turner S, Toone B, Brett-Jones J (1986) Computerised tomographic scan changes in early schizophrenia. Psychol Med 16: 219–225

Van Horn J, McManus I (1992) Ventricular enlargement in schizophrenia. A meta-analysis of studies of the ventricle: brain ratio (VBR). Br J Psychiatry 160: 687–697

Van Os J, Driessen G, Gunther N, Delespaul P (2000) Neighbourhood variation in incidence of schizophrenia — evidence for person-environment interaction. Br J Psychiatry 176: 243–248

Velakoulis D, Phillips U, McGorry PD, Young A, Yuen HP, Brewer WJ, Pantelis C (2000) Larger left hippocapal volume predicts transition to psychosis in an ultra high-risk group. Schizophr Res 41: 117

Verdoux H, Geddes JR, Takei N, Lawrie SM, Bovet P, Eagles JM, Heun R, McCreadie RG, McNeil TF, O'Callaghan E, Stober G, Willinger U, Wright R, Murray RM (1997) Obstetric complications and age at onset in schizophrenia: an international collaborative meta-analysis of individual patient data. Am J Psychiatry 154: 1220–1227

Vita A, Dieci M, Giobbio GM, Tenconi F, Invernizzi G (1997) Time course of cerebral ventricular enlargement in schizophrenia supports the hypothesis of its neurodevelopmental nature. Schizophr Res 23(1): 25–30

Waddington JL, Yuossef HA, Kinsella A (1995) Sequential crosssectional and 10-year prospective study of severe negative symptoms in relation to duration of initially untreated psychosis in chronic schizophrenia. Psychol Med 25: 849–857

Walker EF (1993) Neurodevelopmental aspects of schizophrenia. Schizophr Res 9: 151–152

Walker EF, Lewine RRJ, Neumann C (1996) Childhood behavioural characteristics and adult brain morphology in schizophrenia. Schizophr Res 22: 93–101

Webster MJ, O'Grady J, Orthmann C, Weickert C (2000) Decreased glucocorticoid receptor mRNA levels in individuals with depression, bipolar disorder and schizophrenia. Schizophr Res 41: 111

Weinberger D (1987) Implications of normal brain development for the pathogenesis of schizophrenia. Arch Gen Psychiatry 44: 660–669

Weinberger DR (1995) From neuropathology to neurodevelopment. Lancet 346: 552–557

Weinberger DR, Cannon-Spoor E, Potkin SG, Wyatt RJ (1980) Poor premorbid adjustment and CT scan abnormalities in chronic schizophrenia. Am J Psychiatry 137: 1410–1413

Weinberger DR, DeLisi LE, Perman GP, Targum SD, Wyatt RL (1982) CT scans in schizophreniform disorder and other acute psychiatric patients. Arch Gen Psychiatry 37: 778–783

Weinberger DR, Wagner RL, Wyatt RL (1983) Neuropathological studies of schizophrenia: a selective review. Schizophr Bull 9: 193–212

Westergaard T, Mortensen PB, Pedersen CB, Wohlfahrt J, Melbye M (1999) Exposure to prenatal and childhood infections and the risk of schizophrenia — suggestions from a study of sibship characteristics and influenza prevalence. Arch Gen Psychiatry 56: 993–998

Woodruff P, Murray R (1994) The aetiology of brain abnormalities in schizophrenia. In: Chichester A (ed) Schizophrenia: exploring the spectrum of psychosis. Wiley, Chichester, pp 95–144

Woods BT (1998) Is schizophrenia a progressive neurodevelopmental disorder? Toward a unitary pathogenetic mechanism. Am J Psychiatry 155: 1661–1670

Wright IC, Sharma T, Ellison ZR, McGuire PK, Friston KJ, Brammer MJ, Murray RM, Bullmore ET (1999) Supra-regional brain systems and the neuropathology of schizophrenia. Cereb Cortex 9: 366–378

Wright IC, Rabe-Hesketh S, Woodruff PW, David AS, Murray RM, Bullmore ET (2000) Meta-analysis of regional brain volumes in schizophrenia. Am J Psychiatry 157: 16–25

Wyatt RI (1991) The effect of early neuroleptic intervention on the course of schizophrenia (abstract). Schizophr Res 4: 297

Young KA, Manaye KF, Liang CL, Hicks PB, German DC (2000) Reduced number of mediodorsal and anterior thalamic neurons in schizophrenia. Biol Psychiatry 47(11): 944–953

Zipursky RB, Lim KO, Sullivan EV, Brown BW, Nefferbaum A (1992) Widespread cerebral gray matter volume deficits in schizophrenia. Arch Gen Psychiatry 49: 195–205

Zornberg GL, Buka SL, Tsuang MT (2000) Hypoxic-ischemia-related foetal/neonatal complications and risk of schizophrenia and other nonaffective psychoses: a 19-year longitudinal study. Am J Psychiatry 157: 196–202

Authors' address: Dr. S. M. Church, Department of Psychological Medicine, Institute of Psychiatry, De Crespigny Park, London SE5 8AF, United Kingdom, e-mail: s.church@iop.kcl.ac.uk

Springer-Verlag
and the Environment

GPSR Compliance

The European Union's (EU) General Product Safety Regulation (GPSR) is a set of rules that requires consumer products to be safe and our obligations to ensure this.

If you have any concerns about our products, you can contact us on ProductSafety@springernature.com

In case Publisher is established outside the EU, the EU authorized representative is:

Springer Nature Customer Service Center GmbH
Europaplatz 3
69115 Heidelberg, Germany

Batch number: 10731347

Printed by Printforce, the Netherlands